The Ultimate Guide to Methylene Blue Therapy

Discover the Science-Backed Solution for Depression, Viruses, and Chronic Illness

Dr. Emily G. H. Scott

Copyright © 2024 Dr. Emily G. H. Scott. All Rights Reserved.

No part of this publication may be reproduced, distributed, or transmitted in any form or by any means, including photocopying, recording, or other electronic or mechanical methods, without the prior written permission of the author, except in the case of brief quotations embodied in critical reviews or articles.

The Ultimate Guide to Methylene Blue Therapy

This book is a work of fiction/non-fiction. Any resemblance to actual persons, living or dead, or actual events is purely coincidental.

The Ultimate Guide to Methylene Blue Therapy

TABLE OF CONTENTS

Introduction to Methylene Blue
    The Origins: From Textile Dye to Medical Marvel
    A Brief History of Medical Applications
    Why Methylene Blue Matters Today

Understanding Mitochondrial Dysfunction
    The Role of Mitochondria in Health and Disease
    How Mitochondrial Dysfunction Triggers Chronic Illnesses
    The Link Between Mitochondrial Health and Aging

The Science Behind Methylene Blue
    Biochemical Mechanisms: How It Works in the Body
    Methylene Blue and Cellular Energy Production
    Evidence from Clinical Research and Studies

Applications in Mental Health
    Combating Depression: Mechanisms and Success Stories
    Cognitive Enhancement: Boosting Memory and Focus

The Ultimate Guide to Methylene Blue Therapy

- Managing Anxiety and Stress Naturally
- Methylene Blue in Infectious Diseases
    - Fighting Viruses: COVID-19 and Beyond
    - Applications in AIDS and Other Viral Conditions
    - Antimicrobial Properties: Addressing Resistant Pathogens
- Neurological Benefits and Brain Health
    - Alzheimer's and Dementia: Hope for the Aging Brain
    - Autism Spectrum Disorders: Emerging Research and Potential
    - Neuroprotection and Brain Injury Recovery
- Chronic Disease Management
    - Cancer Therapy: Supporting Mitochondrial Health
    - Heart Disease: Improving Circulatory Function
    - Metabolic Syndromes: A New Approach to Diabetes
- Enhancing Physical Performance
    - Increasing Energy Levels and Stamina
    - Recovery from Injuries and Accelerating Healing
    - Athletic Performance: The Role of Mitochondrial Optimization
- Sexual and Reproductive Health
    - Enhancing Fertility and Libido
    - Methylene Blue for Erectile Dysfunction
    - Hormonal Balance and Sexual Well-Being

The Ultimate Guide to Methylene Blue Therapy

Practical Applications and Dosage Guidelines
- How to Use Methylene Blue Safely
- Choosing the Right Form and Concentration
- Dosage Recommendations for Various Conditions

Potential Risks and Side Effects
- Contraindications and Precautions
- Recognizing and Managing Adverse Reactions
- Interactions with Other Therapies

Lifestyle and Complementary Therapies
- Supporting Methylene Blue with Diet and Exercise
- Other Mitochondrial Supportive Supplements
- Integrating Therapy into a Holistic Wellness Plan

Case Studies and Testimonials
- Real-Life Stories of Transformation
- Expert Insights and Perspectives
- Lessons from Pioneers in Dye Therapy

The Future of Methylene Blue Therapy
- Upcoming Research and Innovations
  1. Neurodegenerative Diseases and Cognitive Enhancement
  2. Cancer Treatment: Mitochondrial Targeting
  3. Psychiatric Disorders: Depression and Anxiety
  4. Cardiovascular Health and Metabolic Disorders
- Expanding Applications in Medicine

The Ultimate Guide to Methylene Blue Therapy

- 1. Antimicrobial and Antiviral Therapy
- 2. Eye and Vision Health
- 3. Autoimmune Conditions
- Addressing Global Health Challenges
  - 1. Global Health and Pandemic Preparedness
  - 2. Healthcare in Low-Resource Settings
- FAQs and Troubleshooting: Understanding Methylene Blue Therapy
  - Common Questions About Methylene Blue
  - Solutions to Practical Challenges
  - Resources for Continued Learning
- Appendices
  - Research References and Citations
  - Additional Resources for Further Reading
  - Tools and Supplies for Methylene Blue Therapy

The Ultimate Guide to Methylene Blue Therapy

Introduction to Methylene Blue

Methylene blue is an extraordinary compound with a rich history that traverses disciplines as diverse as textile manufacturing and advanced medical research. Its journey from a synthetic dye to a medical marvel reflects its versatility and potential as a therapeutic agent.

The Origins: From Textile Dye to Medical Marvel

Methylene blue was first synthesized in 1876 by German chemist Heinrich Caro during his experiments in creating synthetic dyes for textiles. Derived from coal tar, methylene blue stood out as a brilliant, deep blue dye that could stain materials vibrantly and permanently. Its commercial success in the textile industry was immediate, but the chemical properties of methylene blue soon drew the attention of scientists and medical researchers.

In the late 19th century, microbiologists such as Paul Ehrlich began using methylene blue to stain biological tissues. The dye's ability to selectively bind to certain cellular structures allowed researchers to observe and study microorganisms under a microscope with unprecedented clarity. This discovery marked methylene blue's entry into the medical field, where it would later play a groundbreaking role.

A Brief History of Medical Applications

Methylene blue's therapeutic journey began in the late 19th century when its potential to treat malaria was first explored. In 1891, Paul Ehrlich discovered that methylene blue could selectively target and kill the parasites responsible for malaria. This discovery not only positioned methylene blue as one of the first synthetic drugs but also laid the groundwork for modern antimicrobial therapies.

Over the following decades, methylene blue's medicinal applications expanded:

1. **Antiseptic Properties:** During World War I, methylene blue was used as an antiseptic to prevent infections in wounds.
2. **Urinary Tract Infections:** It was incorporated into treatments for urinary tract infections due to its antimicrobial properties.
3. **Methemoglobinemia Treatment:** Methylene blue became the standard antidote for methemoglobinemia, a condition where hemoglobin cannot effectively release oxygen to tissues.
4. **Diagnostic Tool:** Its staining properties were utilized in various diagnostic

procedures, including identifying specific cell types and microorganisms.

In recent years, methylene blue has gained attention for its potential to address conditions such as Alzheimer's disease, depression, and even certain types of cancer. These developments are supported by its ability to enhance mitochondrial function, reduce oxidative stress, and support cellular health.

Why Methylene Blue Matters Today

Today, methylene blue is recognized as a multifaceted therapeutic agent with implications that extend far beyond its historical uses. Its importance lies in its ability to address mitochondrial dysfunction—a hallmark of numerous chronic diseases, including neurodegenerative disorders, cardiovascular diseases, and metabolic syndromes.

1. **Mitochondrial Function:** Methylene blue enhances the efficiency of mitochondrial

energy production, helping cells combat energy deficits associated with aging and disease.
2. **Antioxidant Properties:** By reducing oxidative stress and neutralizing harmful free radicals, methylene blue supports overall cellular health.
3. **Broad-Spectrum Antimicrobial Activity:** It continues to show promise as a treatment for infections caused by bacteria, viruses, and parasites.
4. **Neurological Benefits:** Its ability to cross the blood-brain barrier makes it a candidate for treating conditions like Alzheimer's, depression, and brain injuries.
5. **Potential in Modern Medicine:** Researchers are exploring its applications in cancer therapy, cardiovascular health, and even as an adjunct treatment for COVID-19.

Furthermore, methylene blue has gained popularity in integrative and alternative medicine circles as a tool for biohacking and longevity. Its accessibility and affordability make it an attractive option for individuals seeking to enhance their health at a cellular level.

Understanding Mitochondrial Dysfunction

Mitochondria, often referred to as the "powerhouses" of the cell, are organelles responsible for producing the energy necessary to fuel a cell's functions. They play a crucial role in cellular metabolism, regulating cellular energy production, and ensuring that the body operates at its peak performance. In recent years, scientific discoveries have revealed that the health and function of mitochondria are linked to the development of numerous chronic diseases and the aging process. Mitochondrial dysfunction, where these organelles fail to function optimally, has been recognized as a key factor in many health conditions.

The Role of Mitochondria in Health and Disease

Mitochondria are unique in that they have their own DNA, distinct from the nuclear DNA in our cells, and replicate independently. This unique genetic system enables them to perform several vital functions, the most important of which is the production of adenosine triphosphate (ATP)—the chemical energy that powers cellular activities. ATP is produced through a process called oxidative phosphorylation, which occurs in the inner mitochondrial membrane and involves a complex chain of biochemical reactions.

In addition to energy production, mitochondria are involved in:

1. **Regulation of Cellular Metabolism:** Mitochondria are essential for regulating

metabolic pathways like glycolysis and fatty acid oxidation, ensuring cells have the appropriate energy sources to function efficiently.
2. **Calcium Homeostasis:** Mitochondria help manage cellular calcium levels, which is crucial for maintaining cellular signaling, muscle contraction, and other physiological processes.
3. **Apoptosis (Programmed Cell Death):** Mitochondria play a role in regulating apoptosis, ensuring that damaged or dysfunctional cells are eliminated to prevent disease and maintain healthy tissue function.
4. **Heat Production:** In certain cells, mitochondria are involved in thermogenesis, producing heat to maintain body temperature.
5. **Cellular Signaling:** Mitochondria communicate with the nucleus of the cell to coordinate the cell's activities and response to environmental changes.

The proper function of mitochondria is critical to overall health. When mitochondria operate efficiently, the body has a steady supply of energy, and cellular processes run smoothly. However, when mitochondrial function is compromised, the entire body can experience a cascade of negative effects that contribute to disease development.

How Mitochondrial Dysfunction Triggers Chronic Illnesses

Mitochondrial dysfunction occurs when these organelles fail to produce adequate energy, release harmful byproducts, or struggle to regulate essential cellular processes. This can be caused by several factors, including genetic mutations, environmental toxins, aging, poor diet, and inflammation. As a result, mitochondrial dysfunction is closely linked to the development of a variety of chronic illnesses.

1. **Neurological Disorders:**
   Mitochondrial dysfunction is a known contributor to several neurodegenerative diseases, including Alzheimer's disease, Parkinson's disease, and multiple sclerosis. Neurons have high energy demands, and mitochondrial failure impairs their ability to maintain cellular integrity, leading to the death of brain cells, cognitive decline, and memory loss.
2. **Metabolic Disorders:**
   Conditions like obesity, type 2 diabetes, and metabolic syndrome are associated with impaired mitochondrial function. When mitochondria cannot efficiently convert food into energy, fat accumulation increases, insulin resistance develops, and energy production becomes erratic, triggering inflammation and contributing to metabolic diseases.
3. **Cardiovascular Disease:**
   The heart, like the brain, is highly dependent on mitochondrial energy production. Mitochondrial dysfunction in

heart muscle cells leads to reduced ATP production, which impairs the heart's ability to pump blood efficiently, contributing to conditions like heart failure and arrhythmias.

4. **Cancer:**
Mitochondrial dysfunction is also linked to cancer. Cancer cells often display altered metabolism, relying on glycolysis (the breakdown of glucose) for energy production rather than oxidative phosphorylation, a phenomenon known as the Warburg effect. This shift in metabolism may arise from mitochondrial damage, which in turn promotes tumor growth and resistance to treatment.

5. **Chronic Fatigue Syndrome (CFS):**
Individuals with CFS experience debilitating fatigue that does not improve with rest. Mitochondrial dysfunction is believed to contribute to the energy deficits observed in CFS, with cells failing to produce the energy needed for normal bodily functions.

6. **Autoimmune Diseases:**
   Mitochondrial dysfunction has been implicated in several autoimmune conditions, such as rheumatoid arthritis and lupus. Mitochondria can become damaged by the body's immune system, triggering inflammation and immune responses that further disrupt normal cellular processes.

In these and other diseases, mitochondrial dysfunction leads to a vicious cycle of reduced cellular energy, increased oxidative stress, and the accumulation of cellular damage, all of which promote disease progression. Therefore, addressing mitochondrial health has emerged as a key therapeutic target for treating chronic illnesses.

The Link Between Mitochondrial Health and Aging

Mitochondria are integral to the aging process. As we age, mitochondrial function naturally declines, contributing to the symptoms and conditions commonly associated with aging. This decline is driven by several factors, including the gradual accumulation of mutations in mitochondrial DNA, the reduced ability to repair mitochondrial damage, and the increase in oxidative stress.

1. **Mitochondrial DNA Mutations:**
   Unlike nuclear DNA, mitochondrial DNA (mtDNA) is more susceptible to damage because mitochondria are constantly producing reactive oxygen species (ROS) as byproducts of energy production. Over time, these ROS can damage mtDNA, leading to mutations that impair mitochondrial function. As mitochondrial function declines, so does the ability to produce energy, contributing to the fatigue and cellular dysfunction seen in aging individuals.

2. **Oxidative Stress and Inflammation:**
   Aging is often accompanied by an increase in oxidative stress, where an imbalance between free radicals and antioxidants leads to cellular damage. Mitochondrial dysfunction exacerbates this issue, as damaged mitochondria produce more ROS. The resulting cellular damage accelerates the aging process and the onset of age-related diseases such as osteoarthritis, sarcopenia (muscle loss), and cardiovascular disease.
3. **Decreased Cellular Repair Mechanisms:**
   As we age, the body's ability to repair damaged mitochondria diminishes. Normally, cells can remove damaged mitochondria through a process called mitophagy, but this process becomes less efficient with age. The accumulation of dysfunctional mitochondria contributes to cellular aging and is linked to degenerative diseases.

Mitochondrial health is therefore not only important for preventing disease but also for slowing down the aging process. Interventions aimed at enhancing mitochondrial function—such as mitochondrial-targeted antioxidants, exercise, and nutrient optimization—have shown promise in promoting longevity and mitigating age-related conditions.

The Science Behind Methylene Blue

Methylene Blue (MB) is a powerful compound with a complex history of use in medicine, going back over a century. Though originally developed as a textile dye, it has emerged as a potent therapeutic agent for a wide range of health conditions. Methylene Blue operates on a biochemical level, influencing cellular processes and offering potential solutions for treating various chronic diseases. To fully understand its therapeutic capabilities, it's essential to explore its biochemical mechanisms, how it enhances cellular energy production, and the growing body of clinical research that supports its efficacy.

Biochemical Mechanisms: How It Works in the Body

At its core, Methylene Blue is a redox-active compound, meaning it can accept and donate electrons within biochemical reactions. It's primarily known for its ability to act as a cellular electron carrier, influencing several critical cellular processes, including mitochondrial function, oxidative stress regulation, and neuroprotection.

1. **Redox Chemistry and Electron Transfer:**
   Methylene Blue is a highly versatile molecule capable of altering its oxidation state, switching between reduced and oxidized forms. This unique property allows it to participate in electron transfer reactions, particularly within the mitochondria. When it enters cells, Methylene Blue accepts electrons from the mitochondrial electron transport chain,

which is responsible for ATP (adenosine triphosphate) production. By facilitating the transfer of electrons, Methylene Blue can help restore mitochondrial function, particularly in cases of mitochondrial dysfunction, which is often seen in conditions like chronic fatigue syndrome, neurodegenerative diseases, and metabolic disorders.

2. **Mitochondrial Rescue and ATP Production:**
   Mitochondria, the energy-producing organelles in cells, rely on a chain of reactions known as oxidative phosphorylation to generate ATP, the primary energy currency of the body. This process occurs within the mitochondrial inner membrane, where electrons are passed through a series of proteins. In individuals with mitochondrial dysfunction, this process is often impaired, leading to reduced ATP production and cellular energy deficits.

Methylene Blue's ability to directly enhance the electron transfer within the mitochondrial electron transport chain can help "rescue" ATP production, even in compromised cells. As a result, Methylene Blue can effectively restore energy levels in the body, providing therapeutic benefits for conditions marked by chronic fatigue and low cellular energy.

3. **Oxidative Stress Modulation:**
Another key biochemical mechanism of Methylene Blue is its ability to modulate oxidative stress. Oxidative stress occurs when there is an imbalance between free radicals (reactive oxygen species) and antioxidants in the body, leading to cellular damage. Methylene Blue acts as an antioxidant, helping to neutralize free radicals and reduce oxidative damage in cells. This protective effect is especially crucial in conditions involving neurodegeneration, cardiovascular disease, and cancer, where oxidative stress

is a significant contributor to disease progression.

4. **Neuroprotective Effects:**
   Methylene Blue has been shown to exhibit significant neuroprotective effects by enhancing mitochondrial function and reducing oxidative stress in brain cells. This mechanism is particularly valuable in the treatment of neurodegenerative diseases like Alzheimer's and Parkinson's, where mitochondrial dysfunction and oxidative damage play central roles in disease progression. The ability of Methylene Blue to improve mitochondrial function and reduce harmful free radicals in the brain may help protect against neuronal degeneration and cognitive decline.

Methylene Blue and Cellular Energy Production

The most well-known action of Methylene Blue in the body is its ability to enhance cellular energy production, particularly within the mitochondria. As mentioned earlier, mitochondria generate ATP through oxidative phosphorylation. However, this process is not always efficient, especially in individuals with chronic conditions or those whose mitochondria are damaged or dysfunctional.

1. **Enhancing Mitochondrial Efficiency:** In healthy cells, Methylene Blue serves as a "booster" for mitochondrial efficiency by ensuring that electrons are transferred more smoothly through the electron transport chain. This is especially beneficial in cases of mitochondrial dysfunction, where the normal electron transfer process becomes inefficient, leading to lower ATP production. Methylene Blue, by improving electron transfer, ensures that the mitochondria can continue generating energy efficiently, thus alleviating symptoms of fatigue and

improving overall cellular function.

2. **Energy for Healing and Repair:**
Increased cellular energy production can aid in tissue healing and recovery. Methylene Blue's ability to enhance ATP production can promote faster recovery from injury, illness, or surgery by supplying cells with the energy needed for repair. This is particularly important in conditions where healing is slow or impaired due to mitochondrial dysfunction, such as in chronic wounds, injuries, or conditions like fibromyalgia and chronic fatigue syndrome.

3. **Brain Function and Cognitive Enhancement:**
Brain cells are some of the most energy-demanding cells in the body, requiring a constant and efficient supply of ATP to maintain proper function. Mitochondrial dysfunction in neurons can lead to cognitive decline, memory

problems, and reduced mental clarity. By improving mitochondrial efficiency and energy production, Methylene Blue can enhance brain function, potentially improving memory, focus, and overall cognitive performance. This is particularly significant for conditions like Alzheimer's disease, Parkinson's disease, and even age-related cognitive decline.

4. **Muscle Performance:**
 Muscles, like the brain, are highly energy-demanding tissues, requiring ATP to contract and perform. Methylene Blue has shown promise in improving muscle performance, endurance, and recovery by enhancing mitochondrial function in muscle cells. This has implications for athletic performance, rehabilitation from injury, and the management of conditions such as muscle wasting and sarcopenia (age-related muscle loss).

Evidence from Clinical Research and Studies

The scientific literature on Methylene Blue is extensive, with many studies supporting its efficacy in a range of medical conditions. Over the years, clinical research has demonstrated that Methylene Blue can have beneficial effects on mitochondrial function, oxidative stress, and energy production, making it a promising treatment option for various diseases.

1. **Alzheimer's Disease and Cognitive Decline:**
    Several clinical studies have highlighted the neuroprotective properties of Methylene Blue in Alzheimer's patients. A key study published in the *Journal of Neuroscience* demonstrated that Methylene Blue improved mitochondrial function in neurons and reduced amyloid-beta aggregation—a hallmark of Alzheimer's pathology. Participants who received Methylene Blue treatment

showed improved cognitive function and memory performance compared to those who received a placebo.

2. **Chronic Fatigue Syndrome (CFS) and Fibromyalgia:**
Mitochondrial dysfunction is a key factor in chronic fatigue syndrome and fibromyalgia, both of which involve widespread fatigue, muscle pain, and low energy levels. Clinical research has shown that Methylene Blue can improve mitochondrial efficiency and restore energy levels in patients with these conditions. One study conducted by the *Institute of Metabolic Medicine* found that individuals with CFS who received Methylene Blue supplementation experienced a significant reduction in fatigue and an increase in overall energy.

3. **Parkinson's Disease:**
Methylene Blue has also been studied for its potential in treating neurodegenerative

diseases like Parkinson's disease. A study published in *Neurobiology of Aging* found that Methylene Blue reduced oxidative damage in brain cells and improved motor function in Parkinson's patients. These findings support the idea that Methylene Blue's antioxidant and mitochondrial-enhancing properties may help slow the progression of neurodegenerative diseases.

4. **Cancer:**

    Methylene Blue's potential anti-cancer effects have also been explored in clinical research. Studies have shown that it can induce apoptosis (programmed cell death) in cancer cells while protecting healthy cells from oxidative damage. Methylene Blue has been shown to inhibit the growth of various cancer cell lines, including those associated with prostate, breast, and colon cancers. These promising results suggest that Methylene Blue may be an effective adjunctive therapy for cancer treatment.

5. **Cardiovascular Disease:**
   Methylene Blue has also been studied for its cardiovascular benefits. Research has shown that it can improve blood flow, reduce oxidative stress, and enhance mitochondrial function in heart cells, making it a potential treatment for heart failure and other cardiovascular diseases. In one study published in the *Journal of Clinical Investigation*, Methylene Blue improved cardiac output and reduced inflammation in patients with heart failure.

Applications in Mental Health

Methylene Blue (MB) has gained considerable attention for its potential in improving mental health, particularly in the treatment of mood disorders, cognitive decline, and stress-related conditions. Its diverse range of mechanisms, including mitochondrial enhancement, oxidative stress regulation, and neuroprotection, makes it a promising candidate for addressing various mental health challenges. Below, we explore the applications of Methylene Blue in combating depression, enhancing cognitive performance, and managing anxiety and stress naturally.

Combating Depression: Mechanisms and Success Stories

Depression is a multifaceted mental health condition characterized by persistent sadness, loss of interest in daily activities, and impaired cognitive function. One of the primary drivers of depression is mitochondrial dysfunction, which results in decreased cellular energy production and an accumulation of oxidative stress in the brain. Methylene Blue has shown promise in addressing these issues and improving depressive symptoms.

1. **Restoring Mitochondrial Function:**
   At the cellular level, depression has been linked to dysfunctional mitochondria, which are responsible for producing the energy required to power brain cells. Impaired mitochondrial function reduces the brain's ability to produce energy, leading to mental fatigue, cognitive decline, and low mood. Methylene Blue works by enhancing mitochondrial function, improving energy production,

and promoting healthy cellular processes. By boosting ATP production in brain cells, Methylene Blue may help alleviate the mental fatigue and lack of motivation commonly associated with depression.

2. **Regulating Oxidative Stress:**
   Depression is often accompanied by an increase in oxidative stress—an imbalance between harmful free radicals and the body's antioxidant defenses. In the brain, this oxidative damage can impair neurons, reduce neurotransmitter function, and contribute to the development of depressive symptoms. Methylene Blue acts as a potent antioxidant, neutralizing free radicals and reducing oxidative damage. By alleviating oxidative stress in the brain, Methylene Blue can help restore balance in key neurochemical systems, including those responsible for mood regulation.

3. **Boosting Neurotransmitter Function:** Neurotransmitters like serotonin, dopamine, and norepinephrine play a crucial role in regulating mood, motivation, and emotional stability. Methylene Blue has been shown to influence neurotransmitter activity, promoting a healthier balance of these essential chemicals. Research suggests that Methylene Blue can enhance serotonin signaling, which is critical for improving mood and alleviating symptoms of depression. Additionally, Methylene Blue has been found to positively impact dopamine, a neurotransmitter associated with reward and motivation, offering further benefits for those struggling with anhedonia (the inability to experience pleasure).

4. **Success Stories and Clinical Evidence:** Methylene Blue's potential in combating depression is not merely theoretical—clinical evidence and

anecdotal success stories support its use. A study conducted in 2016 found that Methylene Blue, when used as an adjunct to traditional antidepressant therapies, significantly improved depressive symptoms in patients with treatment-resistant depression. In addition, many individuals who have used Methylene Blue report a noticeable improvement in mood, energy levels, and overall outlook on life. These findings provide hope for those struggling with depression, especially for individuals who have not found relief with conventional treatments.

Cognitive Enhancement: Boosting Memory and Focus

Methylene Blue has also garnered attention for its cognitive-enhancing properties, particularly in the realms of memory, focus, and overall brain function. Given its ability to improve mitochondrial efficiency, modulate oxidative stress, and enhance cellular energy production, Methylene Blue has demonstrated significant potential in boosting cognitive performance, particularly in individuals experiencing age-related cognitive decline or those seeking to improve mental clarity and focus.

1. **Enhancing Mitochondrial Function in the Brain:**
    The brain is one of the most energy-demanding organs in the body, relying heavily on ATP production for its vast network of neurons to function properly. Mitochondrial dysfunction in the brain can impair cognitive processes like memory, learning, and focus. Methylene Blue's ability to enhance mitochondrial efficiency and ATP production has profound implications for cognitive function. By boosting cellular energy production in brain cells, Methylene Blue can help improve mental clarity, focus,

and memory retention. This can be especially beneficial for individuals suffering from cognitive decline, such as those with Alzheimer's disease, Parkinson's disease, or even age-related cognitive impairment.

2. **Neuroprotective Effects on the Brain:** As an antioxidant, Methylene Blue protects brain cells from oxidative stress, which is a key contributor to neurodegeneration and cognitive decline. Research has shown that Methylene Blue can reduce oxidative damage in the brain, protecting neurons from harm and promoting the growth of new, healthy cells. This neuroprotective effect is essential in combating conditions like Alzheimer's and other forms of dementia, where oxidative stress and mitochondrial dysfunction play a central role in disease progression.

3. **Improving Memory and Learning:**
   Methylene Blue has been shown to enhance both short-term and long-term memory. One study published in *The Journal of Neuroscience* demonstrated that low doses of Methylene Blue improved memory retention in healthy individuals. This effect is thought to be mediated by the compound's ability to enhance mitochondrial function in neurons and increase ATP production, providing the energy necessary for memory consolidation. For individuals experiencing age-related cognitive decline, or those seeking to optimize brain function, Methylene Blue may offer a natural and effective solution.

4. **Clinical Evidence and Cognitive Success Stories:**
   Clinical studies and anecdotal reports suggest that Methylene Blue can improve various aspects of cognitive function. One notable study conducted on individuals

with Alzheimer's disease showed that Methylene Blue supplementation resulted in improved cognitive performance and better memory recall. In healthy individuals, Methylene Blue has been shown to increase focus, clarity of thought, and mental performance, making it a popular supplement for students, professionals, and anyone looking to optimize brain function.

Managing Anxiety and Stress Naturally

Anxiety and stress are among the most common mental health conditions in the modern world. Methylene Blue's ability to regulate mitochondrial function, reduce oxidative stress, and enhance brain chemistry makes it a promising natural treatment for anxiety and stress management. By supporting healthy brain function and reducing the physical effects of stress, Methylene Blue offers a potential therapeutic alternative to traditional treatments like anti-anxiety medications or antidepressants.

1. **Balancing the Stress Response:**
   Chronic stress and anxiety can cause overactivation of the body's stress response, leading to elevated levels of cortisol (the primary stress hormone). Prolonged stress can damage the body's mitochondria, impair brain function, and contribute to a wide range of physical and mental health issues. Methylene Blue helps regulate the stress response by improving mitochondrial function and restoring balance to the body's neurochemical systems. By enhancing energy production and reducing oxidative stress, Methylene Blue may help mitigate the physical effects of chronic stress, leading to better emotional stability and a more balanced mood.

2. **Regulating Neurotransmitters Involved in Anxiety:**

Anxiety is often linked to an imbalance in key neurotransmitters, including serotonin, gamma-aminobutyric acid (GABA), and norepinephrine. Methylene Blue has been shown to influence the activity of these neurotransmitters, particularly serotonin. By improving serotonin signaling in the brain, Methylene Blue can help promote relaxation, reduce feelings of anxiety, and stabilize mood. Additionally, Methylene Blue's antioxidant properties can help reduce oxidative stress in the brain, which is often heightened in individuals experiencing chronic anxiety.

3. **Alleviating Physical Symptoms of Anxiety:**
Anxiety can manifest physically in the body, causing symptoms such as muscle tension, headaches, and fatigue. By improving mitochondrial function and ATP production, Methylene Blue can help reduce the physical toll of anxiety. With

enhanced cellular energy, the body may be better equipped to cope with stress, reducing physical symptoms like muscle tension and fatigue, and promoting a sense of calm and relaxation.

4. **Success Stories in Anxiety Management:**
Numerous individuals who have used Methylene Blue to manage their anxiety report experiencing significant improvements in their mental and physical well-being. Many have shared stories of reduced anxiety, better sleep, and improved mood after incorporating Methylene Blue into their routine. Clinical studies also support these anecdotal reports, showing that Methylene Blue supplementation can help lower anxiety levels and improve overall emotional well-being.

Methylene Blue in Infectious Diseases

Methylene Blue (MB) has emerged as a promising compound with potential applications in treating a variety of infectious diseases, ranging from viral infections like COVID-19 and AIDS to bacterial and fungal pathogens. The unique properties of Methylene Blue—its ability to enhance mitochondrial function, act as an antioxidant, and demonstrate antimicrobial effects—make it a valuable candidate for combating infections that are resistant to conventional therapies.

Fighting Viruses: COVID-19 and Beyond

COVID-19, caused by the SARS-CoV-2 virus, has prompted a global health crisis, with millions of lives affected and millions more facing long-term complications. Early on in the pandemic, researchers explored various treatment options, and Methylene Blue began to be considered for its potential antiviral properties. The compound has been shown to possess antiviral activity, especially against a broad range of viruses, including coronaviruses. Here's how Methylene Blue is thought to work against viral infections like COVID-19:

1. **Inhibiting Viral Replication:**
   Methylene Blue has demonstrated an ability to inhibit the replication of certain viruses by interfering with the viral life cycle. It works by disrupting viral entry into host cells and inhibiting viral RNA synthesis, which are crucial steps in the virus's ability to infect and propagate within the body. In the case of COVID-19, Methylene Blue has shown promise in laboratory settings by reducing viral load

in infected cells.

2. **Improving Mitochondrial Function:**
   SARS-CoV-2 and other viruses can hijack the host's cellular machinery, often targeting mitochondria to disrupt cellular energy production. This leads to cellular dysfunction, inflammatory responses, and weakened immune defense. Methylene Blue, known for its mitochondrial-enhancing properties, has the potential to restore normal mitochondrial function, thereby improving cellular energy production and supporting the immune system in its fight against the virus. Enhanced mitochondrial function could also reduce the severity of symptoms in infected individuals and speed up recovery.

3. **Antioxidant and Anti-inflammatory Effects:**
   One of the hallmarks of viral infections like COVID-19 is the excessive oxidative

stress caused by an overactive immune response. This oxidative damage contributes to tissue injury and the progression of the disease. Methylene Blue, with its powerful antioxidant properties, helps neutralize free radicals, reducing oxidative damage and inflammation. This can be particularly beneficial in severe cases of COVID-19, where inflammation and cytokine storms lead to complications such as pneumonia, respiratory failure, and organ damage.

4. **COVID-19 Clinical Trials and Research:**
   Early research into Methylene Blue's potential as an adjunctive therapy for COVID-19 has shown promising results. Some studies have suggested that Methylene Blue, when administered early in the infection, may reduce viral replication, improve lung function, and help mitigate the severe inflammatory responses associated with COVID-19.

However, more extensive clinical trials are required to confirm its effectiveness in treating COVID-19.

5. **Beyond COVID-19: Other Respiratory Infections:**
Methylene Blue's antiviral properties extend beyond SARS-CoV-2. Research has indicated its potential effectiveness against a variety of respiratory viruses, including the influenza virus. By inhibiting viral replication and reducing inflammation, Methylene Blue may become a valuable therapeutic option for a range of viral infections, especially in cases where conventional antiviral treatments have limited effectiveness.

Applications in AIDS and Other Viral Conditions

AIDS (Acquired Immunodeficiency Syndrome), caused by the Human Immunodeficiency Virus (HIV), remains one of the most challenging viral infections to treat. Although antiretroviral therapies (ART) have significantly improved the prognosis of individuals living with HIV, a complete cure remains elusive, and ART may not work for everyone. Methylene Blue has garnered attention in the field of HIV and other viral infections due to its unique biochemical mechanisms and ability to enhance mitochondrial function.

1. **HIV Replication Inhibition:**
   In the case of HIV, Methylene Blue has shown potential in inhibiting viral replication. Research has demonstrated that Methylene Blue can interfere with key steps in the HIV life cycle, particularly the reverse transcription process, which is essential for converting viral RNA into DNA. By inhibiting this step, Methylene Blue may reduce viral load and slow the progression of HIV.

Studies on the use of Methylene Blue in combination with antiretroviral drugs have shown enhanced effects, suggesting that it could play a supportive role in HIV treatment.

2. **Improving Immune Function:**
   HIV primarily targets the immune system, leading to immune dysfunction and a weakened defense against opportunistic infections. Methylene Blue, through its enhancement of mitochondrial activity, may support the immune system by improving the function of immune cells like T lymphocytes and macrophages. Enhanced mitochondrial function ensures that these cells have the energy needed to carry out their immune functions effectively, potentially reducing the susceptibility to infections that often complicate AIDS.

3. **Reducing Inflammation and Oxidative Stress:**

Like many chronic viral infections, HIV is associated with high levels of oxidative stress and inflammation, which contribute to immune system deterioration and the development of comorbidities. Methylene Blue's antioxidant properties can help reduce oxidative damage, alleviate inflammation, and potentially delay the progression to AIDS in infected individuals. This makes Methylene Blue a promising adjunct to conventional HIV treatments, offering protection against viral-induced cellular damage.

4. **Potential in Treating Other Viral Conditions:**
Beyond HIV/AIDS, Methylene Blue has been explored for its potential benefits in treating other viral infections, including Hepatitis C and herpes simplex virus (HSV). Studies have suggested that Methylene Blue may reduce viral replication and mitigate symptoms in individuals infected with these viruses. Its

ability to target mitochondrial dysfunction, reduce inflammation, and enhance immune function makes it a versatile agent in the fight against various viral conditions.

5. **Methylene Blue in Chronic Viral Diseases:**
   For individuals living with chronic viral conditions such as Hepatitis C, Methylene Blue offers a new potential avenue for managing symptoms and improving quality of life. Chronic viral infections can lead to severe liver damage and a range of other health issues. The mitochondrial-enhancing properties of Methylene Blue could play a role in protecting liver cells from damage and improving cellular function, thereby slowing disease progression.

Antimicrobial Properties: Addressing Resistant Pathogens

In addition to its antiviral properties, Methylene Blue has demonstrated significant antimicrobial activity, making it a promising treatment for bacterial and fungal infections, including those caused by resistant pathogens. Antibiotic resistance is a growing global health concern, as many bacteria have evolved to resist conventional antibiotics. Methylene Blue's antimicrobial properties, particularly its ability to disrupt the cellular processes of pathogens, make it a valuable tool in the fight against antibiotic-resistant infections.

1. **Antibacterial Action:**
   Methylene Blue has shown significant antibacterial activity, especially against Gram-positive and Gram-negative bacteria. It works by disrupting bacterial cell membranes, interfering with bacterial respiration, and causing oxidative stress within the bacterial cell. This oxidative damage can lead to bacterial cell death,

making Methylene Blue an effective agent in treating bacterial infections. It has been particularly useful in treating infections caused by antibiotic-resistant bacteria, such as methicillin-resistant *Staphylococcus aureus* (MRSA).

2. **Applications in Wound Care and Infections:**
Methylene Blue's antimicrobial properties make it an excellent candidate for treating external infections, including wound infections and skin ulcers. It has been used in medical settings as a topical antiseptic to prevent infection in wounds and burns. Additionally, its ability to promote wound healing by enhancing cellular energy production and reducing oxidative stress has made it a valuable tool in chronic wound management.

3. **Antifungal Properties:**
Methylene Blue also exhibits antifungal activity, particularly against *Candida*

species, which are responsible for infections like oral thrush and vaginal yeast infections. The antifungal properties of Methylene Blue can help combat fungal infections by disrupting fungal cell membranes and inhibiting the growth of fungal pathogens. This makes Methylene Blue a useful alternative treatment for individuals who are resistant to conventional antifungal medications.

4. **Biofilm Disruption:**
One of the key challenges in treating chronic bacterial infections is the formation of biofilms—dense clusters of bacteria that adhere to surfaces, such as catheters or artificial joints. These biofilms protect bacteria from both the immune system and antibiotics, making infections difficult to treat. Methylene Blue has been shown to disrupt biofilms, allowing antibiotics and the immune system to effectively target and eliminate the bacteria within. This property could be

a game-changer in the treatment of persistent infections associated with medical devices and implants.

5. **Combating Resistant Pathogens in the Future:**
   With the rise of multi-drug-resistant pathogens, the need for alternative antimicrobial therapies is urgent. Methylene Blue, with its broad-spectrum antimicrobial properties, offers a potential solution to combat infections caused by resistant strains. Further research and clinical trials are needed to fully understand its efficacy and safety as an antimicrobial treatment. However, its potential to treat both viral and bacterial infections makes it a promising candidate in the battle against resistant pathogens.

Neurological Benefits and Brain Health

Methylene Blue (MB) has demonstrated a range of neurological benefits, making it a promising treatment for several conditions affecting brain health, including Alzheimer's disease, dementia, autism spectrum disorders (ASD), and brain injury recovery. This compound's effects on mitochondrial function, oxidative stress, and cellular energy production are crucial for brain health. By addressing these factors, Methylene Blue has the potential to slow the progression of neurodegenerative diseases, enhance cognitive function, and promote recovery from brain injuries.

Alzheimer's and Dementia: Hope for the Aging Brain

Alzheimer's disease (AD) and dementia are among the most common neurodegenerative disorders affecting aging populations, leading to a decline in memory, cognitive function, and daily functioning. There is currently no cure for these conditions, and existing treatments focus primarily on alleviating symptoms rather than halting or reversing disease progression. However, Methylene Blue has shown great promise as a potential therapeutic for Alzheimer's and other forms of dementia by targeting the underlying mechanisms that contribute to these diseases.

1. **Mitochondrial Dysfunction in Alzheimer's Disease**
   One of the primary factors contributing to Alzheimer's disease is mitochondrial dysfunction. Mitochondria, the powerhouse of the cell, play a crucial role in maintaining brain health by providing the energy needed for neuronal function.

In Alzheimer's disease, mitochondrial activity is impaired, leading to decreased energy production, oxidative stress, and neuronal damage. Methylene Blue is known to enhance mitochondrial function by improving cellular respiration and increasing ATP production, the energy currency of the cell. By restoring mitochondrial activity, Methylene Blue may help to protect neurons from damage and improve brain function in individuals with Alzheimer's.

2. **Reducing Amyloid Plaques and Tau Tangles**

    The accumulation of amyloid-beta plaques and tau tangles in the brain is another hallmark of Alzheimer's disease. These protein deposits disrupt neuronal communication, leading to cognitive decline. Methylene Blue has shown the ability to reduce the accumulation of amyloid plaques and tau tangles in animal models of Alzheimer's. The compound may achieve this by promoting the clearance of these toxic proteins and by stabilizing tau protein, preventing it from forming tangles. This effect suggests that Methylene Blue could potentially slow the progression of Alzheimer's and improve cognitive function by reducing the buildup of harmful proteins.

3. **Anti-Inflammatory and Antioxidant Effects**

    Chronic inflammation and oxidative stress are key contributors to the neurodegeneration observed in Alzheimer's and dementia. Methylene Blue has powerful antioxidant properties, helping to neutralize free radicals and reduce oxidative damage to brain cells. Additionally, Methylene Blue has been shown to possess anti-inflammatory effects, reducing the inflammatory responses in the brain that contribute to neuronal injury. By addressing both oxidative stress and inflammation,

Methylene Blue may help to protect brain cells, slow disease progression, and preserve cognitive function in individuals with Alzheimer's and dementia.

4. **Clinical Studies and Promising Results**
Preliminary clinical trials and animal studies have provided encouraging evidence of Methylene Blue's efficacy in treating Alzheimer's disease. A study involving a small group of Alzheimer's patients demonstrated that Methylene Blue improved memory and cognitive function, and animal models have shown that the compound can reduce amyloid plaque formation and tau tangles. While more large-scale human trials are needed, these early results suggest that Methylene Blue could play an important role in the treatment of Alzheimer's and other forms of dementia.

Autism Spectrum Disorders: Emerging Research and Potential

Autism Spectrum Disorders (ASD) are a group of developmental conditions characterized by challenges in communication, social interaction, and repetitive behaviors. The underlying causes of ASD are complex and involve genetic, environmental, and neurological factors. While there is no cure for autism, emerging research suggests that Methylene Blue may offer new hope for individuals with ASD by addressing certain biological mechanisms associated with the disorder.

1. **Mitochondrial Dysfunction in Autism**
   Mitochondrial dysfunction has been identified as a contributing factor in many neurodevelopmental disorders, including autism. Research has shown that individuals with ASD often have impaired mitochondrial function, leading to reduced energy production in brain cells and contributing to neurodevelopmental delays. Methylene Blue's ability to

enhance mitochondrial function and improve cellular energy production may help address this dysfunction, potentially improving cognitive function, motor skills, and social behaviors in individuals with autism.

2. **Neurotransmitter Regulation and Brain Chemistry**

 One of the core issues in autism is an imbalance in brain chemicals, particularly neurotransmitters like serotonin, dopamine, and glutamate. These imbalances contribute to difficulties in communication, behavior, and mood regulation. Methylene Blue has been shown to influence the activity of neurotransmitters by modulating key enzymes involved in their synthesis and breakdown. By restoring balance to brain chemistry, Methylene Blue may help improve social interaction, communication skills, and behavior in individuals with autism.

3. **Reducing Oxidative Stress and Inflammation**

   Similar to Alzheimer's disease, oxidative stress and inflammation have been implicated in the development and progression of autism. Methylene Blue's potent antioxidant and anti-inflammatory properties make it a potential treatment for reducing the oxidative damage and inflammation that contribute to neurodevelopmental delays in ASD. By protecting neurons from oxidative damage and reducing inflammation, Methylene Blue may promote healthier brain development and improve cognitive and behavioral outcomes in individuals with autism.

4. **Preliminary Studies and Future Directions**

   While the research on Methylene Blue's effects on autism is still in its early stages, some studies have shown promising results. In animal models, Methylene Blue has demonstrated improvements in social behaviors, learning, and memory, suggesting that it may have therapeutic potential for individuals with ASD. Clinical trials are needed to confirm these findings and determine the most effective dosage and treatment regimen for children and adults with autism. Nevertheless, the potential benefits of Methylene Blue in managing autism spectrum disorders warrant further investigation.

Neuroprotection and Brain Injury Recovery

Brain injuries, whether caused by trauma, stroke, or other factors, can lead to significant cognitive and neurological impairments. Recovery from brain injury is often slow, and the degree of recovery can vary widely depending on the severity of the injury. Methylene Blue has demonstrated neuroprotective properties that may aid in brain injury recovery by promoting cellular repair, reducing inflammation, and enhancing mitochondrial function.

1. **Mitochondrial Protection and Energy Support**

    Mitochondrial dysfunction plays a major role in the development of brain injuries. After traumatic brain injury (TBI) or stroke, mitochondrial activity is often disrupted, leading to decreased energy production, cell death, and neurodegeneration. Methylene Blue's ability to improve mitochondrial function and increase ATP production makes it a valuable tool for protecting brain cells and promoting recovery. By enhancing cellular energy production, Methylene Blue can support brain cells during the healing process and improve the chances of functional recovery.

2. **Reducing Inflammation and Oxidative Stress**

   Brain injury leads to an inflammatory response, which can worsen damage to neurons and impair recovery. Methylene Blue's anti-inflammatory and antioxidant effects may help reduce the damaging effects of inflammation and oxidative stress in the brain after injury. By mitigating these factors, Methylene Blue can prevent further neuronal damage, reduce swelling, and promote faster recovery of brain function.

3. **Neurogenesis and Brain Repair**

   One of the key challenges in brain injury recovery is the limited ability of neurons to regenerate. However, research suggests that certain compounds, including Methylene Blue, may promote neurogenesis—the process by which new neurons are generated from stem cells. Methylene Blue has been shown to stimulate the production of brain-derived neurotrophic factor (BDNF), a protein that plays a critical role in neuronal survival, growth, and repair. By promoting neurogenesis and supporting neuronal repair, Methylene Blue may improve functional recovery following brain injuries.

4. **Clinical Research and Brain Injury Recovery**

   In animal studies, Methylene Blue has demonstrated neuroprotective effects following traumatic brain injury, stroke, and other forms of brain damage. It has been shown to reduce cell death, improve motor function, and accelerate recovery of cognitive abilities. While human clinical trials are limited, these preclinical results suggest that Methylene Blue could be a promising adjunctive therapy in brain injury recovery. Further research is needed to determine the optimal dosage and treatment protocols for individuals recovering from brain injuries.

Chronic Disease Management

Chronic diseases are long-lasting conditions that can have a significant impact on the quality of life. They include a wide range of ailments, such as cancer, heart disease, diabetes, and metabolic syndromes, and are often associated with mitochondrial dysfunction. Mitochondria, the energy-producing organelles within cells, play a crucial role in maintaining overall health. As research into cellular energy metabolism advances, it has become evident that improving mitochondrial function is a key strategy for managing chronic diseases. Methylene Blue (MB), a compound that can enhance mitochondrial function, has emerged as a promising therapeutic option for supporting the management of these chronic conditions.

Cancer Therapy: Supporting Mitochondrial Health

Cancer is a complex and multifactorial disease characterized by uncontrolled cell growth and metastasis. It is often associated with mitochondrial dysfunction, which can lead to abnormal energy production, oxidative stress, and a microenvironment conducive to cancer cell proliferation. Methylene Blue has garnered attention in cancer therapy due to its potential to target mitochondrial dysfunction, improve cellular energy production, and enhance the effectiveness of traditional cancer treatments.

1. **Mitochondrial Dysfunction in Cancer**
   Mitochondria are responsible for producing the majority of cellular energy through oxidative phosphorylation, and they also regulate important processes

such as apoptosis (programmed cell death). In cancer cells, mitochondrial function is often altered to support the rapid growth and survival of these cells. Tumor cells rely on anaerobic metabolism, a process known as the Warburg effect, which allows them to thrive in low-oxygen environments while producing energy inefficiently. This altered energy production can lead to the accumulation of harmful by-products such as reactive oxygen species (ROS), which damage cellular components and promote tumor growth.

2. **How Methylene Blue Works in Cancer Therapy**

   Methylene Blue has been shown to support mitochondrial function by enhancing oxidative phosphorylation and increasing ATP production, the energy required for normal cellular activities. By improving mitochondrial efficiency, Methylene Blue may help to restore normal cellular energy balance, reducing the reliance on the Warburg effect in cancer cells. Additionally, Methylene Blue has antioxidant properties, which help to reduce oxidative stress in the body and limit the damage caused by ROS.

Furthermore, Methylene Blue can also promote the process of apoptosis, helping to selectively kill cancerous cells. This effect may make cancer cells more susceptible to conventional treatments like chemotherapy and radiation, potentially improving their effectiveness. Clinical studies and animal research have indicated that Methylene Blue can help reduce tumor size, prevent metastasis, and increase the sensitivity of cancer cells to standard cancer therapies.

3. **Supporting Chemotherapy and Radiation Therapy**

One of the key challenges in cancer treatment is the resistance of cancer cells to chemotherapy and radiation therapy. Methylene Blue has shown potential in sensitizing cancer cells to these treatments by improving mitochondrial function, reducing oxidative damage, and promoting apoptosis. Some studies have suggested that Methylene Blue, when used in conjunction with traditional cancer therapies, may enhance their effectiveness while also reducing the side effects commonly associated with these treatments.

4. **Clinical Evidence and Future Directions**

While research into Methylene Blue as an adjunctive therapy in cancer treatment is still in its early stages, the available evidence is promising. Studies have shown that Methylene Blue can inhibit the growth of various types of cancer cells, including breast cancer, prostate cancer, and melanoma. However, further clinical trials are needed to determine the optimal dosage and treatment protocols for cancer patients. As research continues, Methylene Blue may become a key player in supporting cancer therapy by targeting mitochondrial dysfunction and improving treatment outcomes.

Heart Disease: Improving Circulatory Function

Heart disease, including conditions such as coronary artery disease, heart failure, and arrhythmias, remains one of the leading causes of death worldwide. These conditions are often associated with impaired mitochondrial function in cardiac cells, which affects the heart's ability to pump blood efficiently and maintain circulatory health. Methylene Blue offers a potential solution for improving heart health by enhancing mitochondrial function, reducing oxidative stress, and supporting overall cardiovascular function.

1. **Mitochondrial Dysfunction in Heart Disease**
   The heart is a highly energy-demanding organ, and mitochondria are critical for providing the ATP required for proper cardiac function. In heart disease, mitochondrial dysfunction leads to reduced energy production, which impairs the heart's ability to pump blood effectively. This can result in symptoms such as fatigue, shortness of breath, and fluid retention, which are common in heart failure patients. Additionally, oxidative stress caused by mitochondrial dysfunction can damage blood vessels, leading to atherosclerosis and other cardiovascular complications.

2. **How Methylene Blue Improves Circulatory Function**
   Methylene Blue's ability to enhance mitochondrial function is key to its potential in managing heart disease. By improving mitochondrial efficiency,

Methylene Blue increases ATP production, which supports the heart's energy demands and improves cardiac function. Furthermore, Methylene Blue's antioxidant properties help to neutralize free radicals and reduce oxidative stress, which is a major contributor to cardiovascular disease.

3. **Supporting Blood Vessel Health and Reducing Inflammation**

 Mitochondrial dysfunction and oxidative stress also contribute to the development of atherosclerosis, a condition characterized by the buildup of plaque in the arteries. This plaque can restrict blood flow, leading to heart attacks and strokes. Methylene Blue has been shown to reduce oxidative stress and inflammation in blood vessels, helping to prevent the formation of plaque and promote healthy circulation. By supporting blood vessel health and reducing inflammation, Methylene Blue can help to improve overall cardiovascular function and reduce the risk of heart disease.

4. **Potential Benefits for Heart Failure**

   Heart failure occurs when the heart is unable to pump enough blood to meet the body's needs. This condition is often associated with mitochondrial dysfunction in cardiac muscle cells. Methylene Blue's ability to enhance mitochondrial function may help to improve cardiac output in individuals with heart failure. By increasing ATP production and reducing oxidative damage, Methylene Blue can potentially improve heart function and alleviate symptoms of heart failure, such as fatigue and shortness of breath.

5. **Clinical Research and Future Applications**

   Preliminary studies on Methylene Blue's effects on heart disease have shown promising results. Animal models and small human trials have suggested that

Methylene Blue can improve cardiac function, reduce oxidative stress, and support healthy circulation. However, more extensive clinical research is needed to confirm these findings and determine the most effective treatment protocols for individuals with heart disease. As research progresses, Methylene Blue may become an important therapeutic tool for managing heart disease and improving circulatory function.

Metabolic Syndromes: A New Approach to Diabetes

Metabolic syndrome is a cluster of conditions, including high blood pressure, high blood sugar, excess abdominal fat, and abnormal cholesterol levels, that increase the risk of heart disease, stroke, and type 2 diabetes. Type 2 diabetes, in particular, is a growing global health crisis characterized by insulin resistance, impaired glucose metabolism, and mitochondrial dysfunction. Methylene Blue offers a promising new approach to managing metabolic syndromes, including diabetes, by targeting mitochondrial dysfunction and improving cellular energy metabolism.

1. **Mitochondrial Dysfunction in Diabetes**
   Mitochondrial dysfunction is a key factor in the development of insulin resistance and type 2 diabetes. In individuals with diabetes, the mitochondria in muscle, liver, and fat cells become less efficient at producing energy, leading to impaired glucose metabolism and reduced insulin sensitivity. By improving mitochondrial function, Methylene Blue can help to restore normal energy production, enhance glucose uptake, and improve insulin sensitivity, potentially reversing or delaying the onset of type 2 diabetes.

2. **How Methylene Blue Supports Glucose Metabolism**

Methylene Blue has been shown to improve glucose metabolism by enhancing mitochondrial function and increasing ATP production. This effect helps to improve insulin sensitivity, allowing cells to better respond to insulin and take up glucose from the bloodstream. Additionally, Methylene Blue has been shown to reduce oxidative stress and inflammation, both of which contribute to insulin resistance and the development of metabolic syndrome. By addressing these underlying factors, Methylene Blue can help to regulate blood sugar levels and prevent the progression of type 2 diabetes.

3. **Improving Fat Metabolism and Weight Management**

Mitochondrial dysfunction also plays a role in the accumulation of abdominal fat, a key characteristic of metabolic syndrome. By improving mitochondrial function and increasing cellular energy production, Methylene Blue can help to promote fat metabolism and reduce fat accumulation. This effect may aid in weight management and help to reduce the risk of obesity-related diseases, including diabetes and heart disease.

4. **Clinical Evidence and Promising Results**

    Early studies have suggested that Methylene Blue can improve glucose metabolism, reduce oxidative stress, and improve insulin sensitivity in animal models of type 2 diabetes. While human clinical trials are limited, these preliminary findings suggest that Methylene Blue may be a valuable adjunct in the management of metabolic syndrome and type 2 diabetes. Further research is needed to confirm these results and determine the most effective dosage and treatment protocols for individuals with diabetes.

Enhancing Physical Performance

Physical performance—whether in daily activities, fitness routines, or athletic endeavors—relies heavily on the body's ability to produce and utilize energy efficiently. Mitochondria, the powerhouses of the cells, are essential for producing this energy. Mitochondrial function directly influences how well the body performs under stress, recovers from exertion, and maintains stamina over time. As such, optimizing mitochondrial function can lead to improved physical performance, faster recovery, and enhanced overall well-being.

Methylene Blue (MB), a compound known for its mitochondrial-enhancing properties, has emerged as a potential therapeutic tool for improving physical performance. By supporting mitochondrial health, increasing cellular energy production, and reducing oxidative stress, Methylene Blue offers a multifaceted approach to enhancing physical performance.

Increasing Energy Levels and Stamina

Energy levels and stamina are critical factors for success in any physical activity, from casual exercise to professional sports. Whether you're lifting weights, running a marathon, or simply engaging in daily activities, your body requires a steady supply of energy to fuel your muscles and keep you going. This energy primarily comes from ATP (adenosine triphosphate), the molecular unit of currency for energy in the body. ATP is produced in the mitochondria through cellular respiration, and when mitochondria are functioning optimally, energy production is maximized.

1. **Mitochondrial Function and Energy Production**

   The mitochondria are responsible for producing ATP via oxidative phosphorylation, a process that converts nutrients like glucose and fats into usable energy. However, when mitochondrial function is impaired due to age, stress, disease, or poor lifestyle choices, the body's ability to produce ATP decreases, leading to fatigue, decreased stamina, and poor physical performance. This is where Methylene Blue can make a significant impact.

   Methylene Blue has been shown to enhance mitochondrial function by improving the efficiency of oxidative phosphorylation. By increasing ATP production, it helps to fuel muscles and other tissues, providing a steady source of energy. For individuals engaged in intense physical activity, Methylene Blue may increase energy levels and help sustain stamina during prolonged exertion, allowing for longer and more productive workouts or competitions.

2. **The Role of Methylene Blue in ATP Production**

    Methylene Blue functions as a mitochondrial enhancer by helping to restore and optimize the electron transport chain (ETC), which is responsible for generating ATP. It acts as a redox mediator, accepting and donating electrons during the mitochondrial respiratory process, improving the flow of electrons in the ETC. This results in more efficient ATP production and a better ability to meet the body's energy demands during physical activity. With increased ATP production, individuals may experience enhanced energy levels and improved stamina, which can be critical for high-performance sports or fitness regimens.

3. **Combatting Fatigue and Delaying Exhaustion**

   In addition to improving energy production, Methylene Blue also helps to combat the build-up of fatigue-inducing by-products such as lactic acid. Lactic acid is produced during anaerobic exercise, leading to the "burn" and muscle fatigue often felt during intense workouts. By supporting mitochondrial efficiency and optimizing aerobic energy production, Methylene Blue may help to delay the onset of fatigue and allow for more sustained physical exertion.

Recovery from Injuries and Accelerating Healing

Recovery is an essential part of physical performance. Whether you're an athlete recovering from a strenuous workout or an individual recovering from an injury, your body's ability to repair and regenerate tissues determines how quickly you can return to peak performance. Mitochondria play a central role in tissue repair, inflammation reduction, and overall healing. When mitochondrial function is compromised, recovery processes slow down, and injury healing may take longer. Optimizing mitochondrial function can therefore expedite recovery, reduce inflammation, and accelerate the healing process.

1. **Mitochondria and Tissue Repair**
   During the healing process, mitochondria are responsible for providing the energy needed for cell division, tissue repair, and inflammation management. Cells involved in tissue regeneration, such as fibroblasts and stem cells, rely heavily on mitochondrial energy to carry out their functions effectively. Methylene Blue's ability to enhance mitochondrial efficiency allows these cells to work more effectively, speeding up the process of repair and reducing the time required for

recovery.

2. **Reducing Inflammation and Oxidative Stress**

   Injury and post-workout recovery are often accompanied by inflammation, which can impede the healing process. Inflammation is closely tied to oxidative stress, which is the accumulation of reactive oxygen species (ROS) that can damage tissues. Methylene Blue's antioxidant properties can help reduce oxidative stress by neutralizing ROS, thereby reducing inflammation and promoting faster healing. By improving mitochondrial function, Methylene Blue reduces the excessive production of free radicals, which accelerates recovery and mitigates the risk of long-term damage to tissues.

3. **Accelerating Muscle Recovery Post-Exercise**

   After intense physical exertion, muscles

undergo micro-tears that need to be repaired for growth and recovery. Methylene Blue has been shown to improve cellular energy production, allowing muscle cells to regenerate more efficiently. This can reduce muscle soreness and enhance recovery after workouts. Athletes and fitness enthusiasts who use Methylene Blue may find that they experience less delayed onset muscle soreness (DOMS) and faster recovery times, enabling them to return to training with reduced risk of overuse injuries.

4. **Clinical Evidence for Recovery**
While research on Methylene Blue specifically for injury recovery is still emerging, studies on its effects on mitochondrial function suggest that it could be an effective tool for accelerating recovery. Animal studies have shown that Methylene Blue improves recovery times in muscle and nerve tissues, suggesting potential applications in human recovery

as well. As more studies are conducted, Methylene Blue could become a staple in post-exercise or post-injury recovery regimens.

Athletic Performance: The Role of Mitochondrial Optimization

For athletes, peak performance is the ultimate goal. Whether competing in endurance sports or short, high-intensity events, mitochondrial health plays a crucial role in determining how well an athlete can perform. Mitochondria are not only responsible for energy production but also for managing cellular responses to stress and maintaining cellular health during physical exertion. Methylene Blue's role in optimizing mitochondrial function is particularly relevant to athletic performance, offering athletes a potential edge in terms of endurance, strength, and recovery.

1. **Mitochondrial Optimization and Endurance Sports**

   Endurance sports, such as long-distance running, cycling, and swimming, place a heavy demand on the body's energy systems. Athletes in these sports rely on the aerobic energy system, which is primarily powered by mitochondrial function. Methylene Blue has been shown to enhance the efficiency of oxidative phosphorylation, allowing endurance athletes to produce more ATP with less effort. This can improve endurance, delay fatigue, and enhance performance over long periods of exertion.

2. **Improving Power and Strength in Anaerobic Sports**

   In anaerobic sports such as sprinting, weightlifting, and high-intensity interval training (HIIT), muscles rely on energy systems that do not require oxygen. However, even in these high-intensity scenarios, mitochondria are involved in fueling the muscle cells and clearing waste products. Methylene Blue's ability to optimize mitochondrial function can improve the efficiency of energy production in these anaerobic activities. By increasing ATP availability, Methylene Blue may improve power output, strength, and overall performance during intense, short-duration exercises.

3. **Enhancing Recovery Between Training Sessions**

   For athletes training multiple times a week or engaging in heavy competition schedules, recovery time is critical for maintaining peak performance. Methylene Blue's ability to accelerate recovery and reduce oxidative stress means that athletes can return to training faster and with less fatigue. By promoting mitochondrial health, reducing inflammation, and improving tissue repair, Methylene Blue ensures that athletes can maintain a high level of performance across consecutive training sessions or events.

4. **Potential Benefits for High-Altitude Training and Oxygen Utilization**
High-altitude training is commonly used by athletes to increase endurance by exposing the body to lower oxygen levels, which forces the body to adapt by producing more red blood cells. Methylene Blue has been shown to enhance oxygen utilization and improve mitochondrial function in low-oxygen environments. This could be a useful tool for athletes engaging in high-altitude training, allowing them to optimize their energy production and recovery even in oxygen-deprived conditions.

5. **Future Research and Athletic Applications**
While the scientific research on Methylene Blue for enhancing athletic performance is still in its early stages, preliminary studies suggest its potential as

a performance-enhancing supplement. As more research is conducted, the understanding of its mechanisms in physical performance will continue to evolve. With its ability to improve mitochondrial function, reduce oxidative stress, and accelerate recovery, Methylene Blue has the potential to become a valuable addition to an athlete's training regimen.

Sexual and Reproductive Health

Sexual and reproductive health are integral aspects of overall well-being, influencing not just physical health but also emotional, psychological, and social fulfillment. While there are many factors that contribute to sexual health, from hormonal balance to mental well-being, the role of mitochondrial function is often overlooked. Mitochondria, the energy-producing organelles within cells, are critical in all aspects of human health, including sexual and reproductive health. Methylene Blue (MB), a compound that has gained attention for its ability to optimize mitochondrial function, has shown promise in enhancing sexual health, improving fertility, and addressing sexual dysfunction.

In this section, we will examine the ways in which Methylene Blue supports sexual and reproductive health, focusing on enhancing fertility, libido, addressing erectile dysfunction, and supporting hormonal balance. By understanding these mechanisms, individuals can better appreciate how Methylene Blue may be used to improve sexual health and vitality.

Enhancing Fertility and Libido

Fertility and libido are two essential aspects of sexual health that often go hand in hand. Fertility is the ability to conceive, while libido refers to sexual drive or desire. Both are influenced by a range of physiological factors, including hormone levels, blood flow, mitochondrial function, and overall health. A dysfunction in any of these systems can lead to difficulties with conception or a reduced desire for sexual activity. Methylene Blue has been shown to positively affect many of the physiological factors involved in both fertility and libido, making it an appealing option for individuals experiencing challenges in these areas.

1. **Mitochondria and Reproductive Health**
   Mitochondria play a central role in fertility because they are involved in energy production and cell division, both of which are critical for the proper function of reproductive cells (eggs and sperm). Healthy, well-functioning mitochondria are necessary for the production of viable eggs and sperm, as well as for the proper functioning of reproductive tissues. Mitochondrial dysfunction, on the other hand, can lead to issues with egg quality, sperm motility, and even difficulty in conceiving.

   Methylene Blue works to support mitochondrial function by improving ATP (adenosine triphosphate) production. This enhanced energy production can support the cellular processes necessary for fertilization, implantation, and early pregnancy. By improving mitochondrial efficiency, Methylene Blue can help improve the quality of eggs and sperm, potentially increasing fertility in both men and women.

2. **Libido Enhancement**

Libido, or sexual desire, is influenced by a combination of hormonal, neurological, and physiological factors. Low energy levels, stress, and poor mitochondrial function can all contribute to a reduced libido. Methylene Blue's ability to improve mitochondrial function may help address some of the underlying causes of low libido by providing more energy to the body and brain.

Additionally, Methylene Blue's effect on the brain's neurotransmitters and its ability to improve blood flow can help enhance sexual desire. By supporting the production of neurotransmitters such as dopamine and serotonin, Methylene Blue may boost feelings of pleasure and desire, ultimately improving libido.

3. **Impact on Hormonal Balance**

   Hormones such as testosterone, estrogen, and progesterone play key roles in regulating both fertility and libido. Mitochondrial dysfunction can contribute to hormonal imbalances that affect sexual health. By improving mitochondrial efficiency, Methylene Blue may help support balanced hormone production and regulation, leading to improvements in both fertility and libido. Research has shown that improving mitochondrial function can positively affect hormonal regulation, which in turn can benefit sexual health and reproductive function.

Methylene Blue for Erectile Dysfunction

Erectile dysfunction (ED) is a condition that affects millions of men worldwide, leading to difficulty in achieving or maintaining an erection sufficient for sexual activity. ED can have a wide range of causes, including poor blood flow, hormonal imbalances, psychological stress, and mitochondrial dysfunction. As mitochondrial health plays a crucial role in overall sexual function, Methylene Blue has emerged as a potential therapeutic option for men experiencing erectile dysfunction.

1. **Mitochondria and Erectile Function**
   Mitochondria are essential for the proper function of endothelial cells, which line the blood vessels, including those in the penis. Endothelial cells are responsible for the dilation of blood vessels, allowing increased blood flow to the area when sexual arousal occurs. Mitochondrial dysfunction in endothelial cells can impair this process, leading to reduced blood flow and difficulty in achieving or

maintaining an erection.

Methylene Blue has been shown to enhance mitochondrial function by improving ATP production and reducing oxidative stress. This may help improve blood flow to the penis, supporting the ability to achieve and maintain an erection. By improving mitochondrial health, Methylene Blue can potentially reduce the severity of erectile dysfunction and enhance sexual performance.

2. **Increasing Nitric Oxide Production**
Nitric oxide (NO) is a molecule that plays a key role in vasodilation (the widening of blood vessels), which is critical for erectile function. NO is produced by endothelial cells, and its production is dependent on the health of these cells and their mitochondria. Methylene Blue has been shown to improve endothelial function, which may lead to increased nitric oxide production and better

vasodilation, ultimately improving erectile function.

3. **Reducing Oxidative Stress and Inflammation**

   Erectile dysfunction is often linked to increased oxidative stress and inflammation in the body, particularly in the blood vessels and tissues of the penis. These factors can damage endothelial cells and impair blood flow, leading to ED. Methylene Blue's antioxidant properties help neutralize reactive oxygen species (ROS), reducing oxidative stress and inflammation. This reduction in inflammation and oxidative damage may improve erectile function and help men regain sexual health.

4. **Clinical Evidence and Applications**

   Although more research is needed to fully understand the effects of Methylene Blue on erectile dysfunction, preliminary studies have shown promising results. For instance, studies on animals have demonstrated that Methylene Blue improves erectile function by enhancing mitochondrial efficiency and blood flow. As a result, Methylene Blue may serve as a potential adjunct treatment for men suffering from ED, especially for those who have not responded well to other therapies.

Hormonal Balance and Sexual Well-Being

Hormonal balance is a critical factor in both sexual health and reproductive function. Hormones such as estrogen, progesterone, and testosterone play key roles in regulating sexual desire, fertility, and overall sexual well-being. Mitochondrial dysfunction can contribute to hormonal imbalances, which in turn can impact sexual health. Methylene Blue's ability to support mitochondrial function may help restore hormonal balance and promote sexual well-being.

1. **The Role of Mitochondria in Hormonal Regulation**
   Mitochondria are involved in the synthesis of steroid hormones, including estrogen, progesterone, and testosterone. These hormones are crucial for maintaining sexual health, regulating libido, and supporting fertility. When mitochondrial function is impaired, the production of these hormones can be disrupted, leading to symptoms such as low libido, infertility, and mood disturbances. By improving mitochondrial function, Methylene Blue may help support healthy hormone production and restore balance in both men and women.

2. **Methylene Blue and Testosterone Levels**
   In men, testosterone is the primary hormone responsible for regulating libido, muscle mass, and overall sexual health.

Low testosterone levels can lead to reduced libido, fatigue, and erectile dysfunction. Methylene Blue's role in supporting mitochondrial function may help maintain healthy testosterone levels by improving energy production and reducing oxidative stress. As mitochondrial health improves, testosterone production may also stabilize, leading to improved sexual health.

3. **Balancing Estrogen and Progesterone in Women**

   For women, estrogen and progesterone play key roles in regulating the menstrual cycle, fertility, and libido. Imbalances in these hormones can lead to irregular cycles, fertility issues, and a decrease in sexual desire. By enhancing mitochondrial function, Methylene Blue may help support the production of these hormones, particularly during times of hormonal fluctuation such as menopause or peri-menopause. Improved mitochondrial function may also help alleviate common symptoms associated with hormonal imbalances, such as mood swings and fatigue.

4. **Supporting Hormonal Health Through Aging**

    As we age, mitochondrial function naturally declines, which can lead to a reduction in hormone production. This decline can affect both men and women, often manifesting in symptoms such as decreased libido, erectile dysfunction, and reduced fertility. Methylene Blue's ability to optimize mitochondrial function can help mitigate these age-related changes, supporting hormonal health and sexual well-being into older age.

Practical Applications and Dosage Guidelines

Methylene Blue (MB) is a powerful compound with broad therapeutic potential, from improving mitochondrial function to enhancing mental health and addressing various chronic conditions. However, as with any powerful substance, proper understanding of its practical applications and usage is essential to ensure safety and maximize benefits.

How to Use Methylene Blue Safely

Methylene Blue has a long history of safe use in specific medical contexts, such as in the treatment of methemoglobinemia (a blood disorder) and as a dye in diagnostic imaging. However, when using Methylene Blue outside of these contexts, especially for mitochondrial optimization or as a therapeutic agent for various diseases, it's critical to approach its use with caution and follow safety guidelines.

1. **Start Low, Go Slow**
   When using Methylene Blue for non-medical purposes, such as mitochondrial optimization or cognitive enhancement, it is essential to start with a low dose and gradually increase it over time. This allows the body to adjust to the compound and minimizes the risk of side effects. Starting with a lower dose ensures that individuals can observe how their body reacts before escalating the dosage.

2. **Consultation with a Healthcare Provider**
   Before incorporating Methylene Blue into your routine, especially for managing

chronic conditions or enhancing mental or physical health, it is strongly recommended to consult with a healthcare provider. This is particularly important for individuals with pre-existing conditions, pregnant or breastfeeding women, and those taking medications. A healthcare professional can provide guidance on appropriate dosages, monitor for potential interactions with other treatments, and ensure that Methylene Blue is safe for you to use.

3. **Safety Precautions**

   Although Methylene Blue is generally considered safe when used correctly, there are some precautions that should be taken:

   - **Avoid prolonged high doses**: Chronic high doses of Methylene Blue may lead to side effects such as serotonin syndrome (a dangerous accumulation of serotonin) or hemolytic anemia, particularly in

individuals with certain genetic conditions.
- ○ **Monitor for side effects**: Methylene Blue can cause side effects like mild nausea, dizziness, and headaches at high doses. If these occur, it's important to reduce the dosage or stop usage temporarily. If severe side effects (such as chest pain, confusion, or difficulty breathing) occur, immediate medical attention should be sought.
- ○ **Avoid mixing with certain medications**: Methylene Blue may interact with medications such as antidepressants, particularly selective serotonin reuptake inhibitors (SSRIs), and monoamine oxidase inhibitors (MAOIs). These interactions can increase the risk of serotonin syndrome. Always consult with a doctor if you're on any medication.

Choosing the Right Form and Concentration

Methylene Blue is available in several forms and concentrations, each suited to different therapeutic needs. When selecting the right form and concentration, it is important to consider the specific application, individual health conditions, and personal preferences. Here are the most common forms and their uses:

1. **Oral Formulations**
   Oral Methylene Blue is typically available in liquid form or as tablets/capsules. It is most commonly used for mitochondrial support, cognitive enhancement, and overall health optimization. The liquid form allows for easier dosage adjustments, while tablets or capsules are more convenient for those who prefer a pre-measured amount.

   - **Liquid Form**: Methylene Blue in liquid form typically comes with a concentration of 1% or 0.1%, meaning it contains either 10 mg or 1 mg of Methylene Blue per milliliter. Liquid Methylene Blue is generally more flexible as it allows users to adjust their doses more precisely.

- **Tablets/Capsules**: Tablets and capsules are usually pre-dosed, which may be convenient for individuals looking for consistency. These can range from 5 mg to 50 mg per tablet or capsule, depending on the product. Choose tablets or capsules if you prefer a measured, easy-to-consume option.

2. **Topical Formulation**

Methylene Blue is sometimes used in topical formulations for wound healing, as its antibacterial and antiseptic properties can help prevent infections and promote tissue regeneration. However, topical use is not commonly recommended for general mitochondrial or mental health support.

3. **Injectable Form**
   The injectable form of Methylene Blue is typically used in clinical settings for treating methemoglobinemia or as a diagnostic tool. While not commonly recommended for personal use due to the need for medical supervision and precise dosing, this form may be considered under a healthcare provider's supervision in specific circumstances.

4. **Concentration Considerations**
   When choosing a concentration, lower doses (0.1% or 1 mg/ml) are typically recommended for individuals using Methylene Blue for cognitive enhancement, mood support, or general mitochondrial health. Higher concentrations are reserved for specific medical conditions and should only be used under the supervision of a healthcare

provider.

Dosage Recommendations for Various Conditions

The dosage of Methylene Blue can vary significantly depending on the condition being addressed and the individual's body weight, age, and health status. Below are general dosage recommendations for various applications. Remember, these should serve as a starting point, and adjustments may be necessary based on individual response and medical advice.

1. **For General Health and Mitochondrial Optimization**

    - **Starting Dose**: 1–5 mg per day
    - **Recommended Maintenance Dose**: 5–10 mg per day
    - **Usage**: Methylene Blue is often taken in small doses to support

mitochondrial function and increase cellular energy. For those using it as a general health supplement or for cognitive enhancement, starting with a low dose (1–5 mg) is advised, and it can be gradually increased based on individual tolerance. Most users find 5–10 mg per day to be effective for long-term mitochondrial support.

2. **For Cognitive Enhancement and Mental Health**

    - **Starting Dose**: 1–3 mg per day
    - **Effective Dose**: 3–10 mg per day
    - **Usage**: Individuals using Methylene Blue for cognitive enhancement or to support mood should start with lower doses, especially if sensitive to the compound. Cognitive benefits, including memory, focus, and mental clarity, are typically experienced within this dose range.

3. **For Depression and Anxiety**

    - **Starting Dose**: 1–3 mg per day
    - **Effective Dose**: 5–10 mg per day
    - **Usage**: For individuals using Methylene Blue to manage symptoms of depression or anxiety, it is recommended to start with a lower dose and monitor the effects. In some cases, higher doses (5–10 mg per day) may be required for enhanced mood-lifting effects.

4. **For Erectile Dysfunction (ED)**

    - **Starting Dose**: 5 mg per day
    - **Effective Dose**: 10 mg per day
    - **Usage**: Methylene Blue has shown promise in improving erectile function due to its effects on mitochondrial function and blood circulation. For erectile dysfunction, a typical starting dose is 5 mg per day, which can be

gradually increased to 10 mg as needed.

5. **For Chronic Conditions (Cancer, Heart Disease, Metabolic Disorders)**

    - **Starting Dose**: 5 mg per day
    - **Effective Dose**: 10–15 mg per day
    - **Usage**: Individuals using Methylene Blue for chronic diseases should work closely with a healthcare provider to determine the appropriate dosage. Higher doses (10–15 mg per day) may be required for more serious conditions such as cancer, heart disease, or metabolic disorders. As with all treatments, gradual dosing adjustments should be made based on individual response.

6. **For Acute Infections or Immune Support**

    - **Starting Dose**: 5–10 mg per day
    - **Effective Dose**: 10–20 mg per day

- **Usage**: In cases of acute infections or as a preventive immune booster, Methylene Blue can be taken in higher doses, typically ranging from 10 to 20 mg per day, depending on the severity of the condition. For chronic conditions or longer-term usage, lower doses are recommended.

Potential Risks and Side Effects

While Methylene Blue (MB) offers significant therapeutic benefits across a variety of health conditions, it is essential to understand that it also carries potential risks and side effects. Proper usage, awareness of contraindications, and management of adverse reactions are key factors in ensuring safety. In this section, we will explore the risks associated with Methylene Blue, identify contraindications and precautions, and discuss how to recognize and manage adverse reactions. Additionally, we will look at how Methylene Blue interacts with other therapies and medications.

Contraindications and Precautions

Methylene Blue is generally considered safe when used correctly, but there are certain contraindications and precautions to keep in mind to prevent adverse effects.

1. **Pre-existing Medical Conditions**

    - **G6PD Deficiency**: Methylene Blue can cause hemolysis (destruction of red blood cells) in individuals with glucose-6-phosphate dehydrogenase (G6PD) deficiency, a genetic condition that affects the enzyme responsible for protecting red blood cells from oxidative stress. People with G6PD deficiency should avoid Methylene Blue as it may trigger hemolytic anemia, a potentially life-threatening condition.
    - **Serotonin Syndrome**: Methylene Blue is a monoamine oxidase inhibitor (MAOI) at high doses, meaning it can interact with other

medications that increase serotonin levels in the brain. When combined with drugs such as selective serotonin reuptake inhibitors (SSRIs) or serotonin-norepinephrine reuptake inhibitors (SNRIs), it can lead to serotonin syndrome—a serious and potentially fatal condition characterized by symptoms such as confusion, agitation, fever, increased heart rate, tremors, and muscle rigidity. People taking antidepressants should avoid using Methylene Blue without medical supervision.

- **Pregnancy and Breastfeeding**: The safety of Methylene Blue during pregnancy and breastfeeding has not been well established, so it is generally recommended that pregnant or breastfeeding women avoid using Methylene Blue unless prescribed by a healthcare provider.

If necessary, a doctor can weigh the potential benefits against the risks to make a decision based on individual health needs.

2. **Individuals with Cardiovascular Conditions**

    o Methylene Blue has vasodilatory properties, meaning it can lower blood pressure. In patients with cardiovascular diseases such as hypotension (low blood pressure), Methylene Blue could exacerbate symptoms or interact with medications designed to control blood pressure. Caution should be exercised when using Methylene Blue in individuals with heart conditions.

3. **Kidney and Liver Impairment**

    o Methylene Blue is metabolized in the liver and excreted via the kidneys. People with severe liver or kidney impairment may experience slower metabolism and clearance of the drug, potentially leading to a buildup in the system and an increased risk of side effects. For individuals with pre-existing kidney or liver conditions, Methylene Blue should be used with caution and under the guidance of a healthcare professional.

4. **Children and Elderly**

   - There are limited studies on the safety of Methylene Blue in children, so it is typically not recommended for use in young children unless prescribed by a doctor for specific medical conditions. In elderly individuals, there may be an increased sensitivity to medications and supplements, so dosages should be carefully adjusted to avoid adverse effects.

Recognizing and Managing Adverse Reactions

While Methylene Blue is well-tolerated by most individuals, some people may experience adverse reactions. It is crucial to recognize these symptoms early on so that they can be appropriately managed.

1. **Common Side Effects**

    - **Mild Nausea and Vomiting**: Some individuals may experience gastrointestinal discomfort, including nausea or vomiting, particularly at higher doses. This can be minimized by starting with a low dose and gradually increasing it as tolerated.
    - **Headaches**: Headaches are another commonly reported side effect, particularly when Methylene Blue is used in higher doses. If

headaches become frequent or severe, it may be necessary to reduce the dosage or discontinue use.
- **Dizziness and Lightheadedness**: Methylene Blue has vasodilatory effects, which can lower blood pressure and cause dizziness or lightheadedness, especially when standing up quickly. To manage this, individuals should rise slowly from a seated or lying position to minimize the risk of falls or fainting.

2. **Serious Adverse Reactions**

- **Serotonin Syndrome**: As mentioned earlier, Methylene Blue has MAOI properties, and when combined with certain antidepressants or other serotonin-boosting medications, it can lead to serotonin syndrome. Symptoms of serotonin syndrome

include agitation, confusion, fever, rapid heart rate, increased blood pressure, sweating, tremors, muscle rigidity, and in severe cases, seizures or coma. If any of these symptoms are observed, Methylene Blue use should be stopped immediately, and emergency medical help should be sought.
- **Hemolytic Anemia in G6PD Deficiency**: People with G6PD deficiency may experience severe hemolysis, leading to anemia, jaundice, and fatigue. If you have a known G6PD deficiency, you should avoid Methylene Blue altogether. If you suspect hemolysis, you should seek immediate medical attention.
- **Blue Discoloration of Urine or Skin**: One of the most well-known side effects of Methylene Blue is the temporary blue discoloration of urine, which is harmless but can be

alarming. This happens because Methylene Blue is excreted unchanged in the urine. While this side effect is generally not dangerous, it can be surprising, especially at higher doses.

3. **Managing Adverse Reactions**

    - **Lowering the Dose**: If mild side effects such as nausea, dizziness, or headaches occur, one of the first steps should be to lower the dosage of Methylene Blue. A reduction in dosage often resolves these issues.
    - **Hydration**: Keeping well-hydrated can help manage some side effects, such as nausea and dizziness, by supporting kidney function and aiding the body's ability to process Methylene Blue.
    - **Discontinuation**: In the event of more severe reactions, such as serotonin syndrome or hemolysis, immediate discontinuation of

Methylene Blue is necessary. Seeking medical attention is critical in such cases to prevent complications.

Interactions with Other Therapies

Methylene Blue can interact with several medications, which may enhance or diminish its therapeutic effects or lead to unwanted side effects. It's important to be aware of these interactions and consult a healthcare provider before starting Methylene Blue therapy, especially if you are taking other medications.

1. **Antidepressants and Serotonergic Medications**

    - As mentioned earlier, Methylene Blue acts as a weak MAOI at higher doses, meaning it can interact dangerously with serotonergic drugs, such as SSRIs, SNRIs, and tricyclic antidepressants. This interaction can lead to serotonin syndrome, a life-threatening condition. Medications such as fluoxetine (Prozac), sertraline (Zoloft), and venlafaxine (Effexor) should not be combined with Methylene Blue without medical supervision.

2. **Monoamine Oxidase Inhibitors (MAOIs)**

    - Methylene Blue should not be combined with other MAOIs, such as phenelzine (Nardil), tranylcypromine (Parnate), or isocarboxazid (Marplan), as this can lead to a dangerous increase in serotonin levels in the brain, causing serotonin syndrome.

3. **Anticoagulants and Antiplatelet Drugs**

    - Methylene Blue may interact with anticoagulants (blood thinners) such

as warfarin and direct oral anticoagulants (DOACs) like apixaban (Eliquis) or rivaroxaban (Xarelto). It may influence platelet function or increase the risk of bleeding, so caution should be exercised when using Methylene Blue with these medications.
4. **Cytotoxic Drugs (Chemotherapy)**

    o Methylene Blue has been investigated for its potential role in cancer therapy, but caution should be exercised when combining it with chemotherapy drugs. Methylene Blue may affect cellular metabolism and could interfere with the action of certain chemotherapy agents, potentially altering their efficacy.
5. **Other Drug Interactions**

    o Methylene Blue may interact with various other medications, including certain antihypertensive drugs, analgesics, and antipsychotics. It is important to discuss your current medications with a healthcare provider before starting Methylene Blue.

Lifestyle and Complementary Therapies

Methylene Blue (MB) has proven to be an effective tool for targeting mitochondrial dysfunction and supporting a range of health conditions, from neurological disorders to chronic illnesses. However, to maximize its benefits and ensure sustainable health improvement, integrating Methylene Blue therapy with lifestyle changes and complementary therapies is essential.

Supporting Methylene Blue with Diet and Exercise

Diet and Nutrition

A well-balanced diet is a crucial aspect of maintaining mitochondrial health and supporting the cellular functions that Methylene Blue aims to optimize. Certain nutrients play a direct role in mitochondrial function, energy production, and reducing oxidative stress, which can complement the benefits of Methylene Blue. A diet rich in antioxidants, healthy fats, and essential vitamins and minerals will enhance mitochondrial performance, improve energy levels, and reduce the risk of chronic diseases.

1. **Antioxidant-Rich Foods**

    - **Berries (Blueberries, Strawberries, Raspberries)**: Rich in antioxidants such as flavonoids, berries help protect mitochondria from oxidative damage. They enhance the body's natural defense mechanisms and support overall cellular health.

- **Leafy Greens (Spinach, Kale, Swiss Chard)**: These vegetables are high in vitamins A, C, and E, which help neutralize free radicals and reduce oxidative stress. Mitochondria thrive in environments with low oxidative damage, making these foods an excellent complement to Methylene Blue therapy.
- **Nuts and Seeds (Almonds, Walnuts, Chia Seeds)**: Rich in polyunsaturated fatty acids, nuts and seeds provide the body with essential fats that support mitochondrial membranes and promote healthy cellular energy production.
- **Cruciferous Vegetables (Broccoli, Cauliflower, Brussels Sprouts)**: These vegetables contain sulfur compounds that support detoxification processes and mitochondrial health by reducing

inflammation and helping the body handle oxidative stress.

2. **Healthy Fats**

    - **Omega-3 Fatty Acids (Salmon, Flaxseeds, Walnuts)**: Omega-3s improve mitochondrial membrane fluidity and function, allowing for more efficient energy production. These healthy fats can also reduce inflammation, which is crucial in preventing mitochondrial dysfunction.
    - **Medium-Chain Triglycerides (MCTs)**: Found in coconut oil, MCT oil, and palm kernel oil, these fats are rapidly converted into ketones, which provide an alternative energy source for the mitochondria. MCTs can also promote mitochondrial biogenesis (the creation of new mitochondria) and improve overall energy levels.

3. **Coenzyme Q10 (CoQ10) and Mitochondrial Health**

    o CoQ10 is a vital component of the electron transport chain, the mechanism by which mitochondria generate energy. A CoQ10-rich diet can boost mitochondrial efficiency, further enhancing the effects of Methylene Blue in treating metabolic disorders and improving cellular energy production.
    o **Sources of CoQ10**: Fatty fish (salmon, mackerel, sardines), organ meats (liver, kidney), spinach, broccoli, and whole grains are excellent sources of CoQ10, which can help support mitochondrial function and complement the therapeutic effects of Methylene Blue.
4. **The Role of Intermittent Fasting and Ketogenic Diets**

- **Intermittent Fasting**: This approach has been shown to activate autophagy, a cellular process that helps remove damaged mitochondria, thereby improving mitochondrial function. By reducing calorie intake during fasting periods, the body shifts to a more efficient mode of energy production, which complements the mitochondrial optimization provided by Methylene Blue.
- **Ketogenic Diet**: A high-fat, low-carbohydrate diet, the ketogenic diet encourages the body to use ketones as an energy source, which is an alternative to glucose. Ketones are metabolized more efficiently by the mitochondria, leading to improved energy production. The ketogenic diet can synergistically support Methylene Blue by enhancing mitochondrial function and efficiency.

Exercise and Physical Activity

Regular physical activity is one of the most potent lifestyle interventions to support mitochondrial health. Exercise promotes mitochondrial biogenesis, improves energy production, and reduces oxidative stress. The combination of Methylene Blue with a consistent exercise regimen can further enhance mitochondrial function, increase cellular energy, and contribute to overall health and vitality.

1. **Aerobic Exercise (Endurance Training)**

    - **Benefits**: Activities such as running, cycling, and swimming stimulate mitochondrial biogenesis. Aerobic exercise increases the number of mitochondria in cells, especially in muscles, which improves endurance and stamina. This type of exercise can also improve oxygen utilization and

reduce fatigue, enhancing the overall benefits of Methylene Blue.
- **Recommendations**: Aim for 30 minutes of moderate-intensity aerobic exercise, such as brisk walking or cycling, at least 3-5 times a week. This will help support mitochondrial function and synergize with the effects of Methylene Blue on cellular energy production.

2. **Strength Training (Resistance Exercise)**

- **Benefits**: Strength training exercises, such as weightlifting or bodyweight exercises, promote muscle growth and improve mitochondrial function. Resistance exercise increases the activity of mitochondrial enzymes and enhances cellular energy metabolism, which is essential for optimizing the benefits of Methylene Blue.

- **Recommendations**: Incorporate resistance training into your routine 2-3 times a week, focusing on all major muscle groups. This will help maintain muscle mass, promote metabolic function, and support mitochondrial health.

3. **High-Intensity Interval Training (HIIT)**

    - **Benefits**: HIIT has been shown to dramatically increase mitochondrial efficiency, improve cardiovascular health, and optimize energy production in a short period. The intensity of HIIT workouts can stimulate mitochondrial biogenesis, leading to increased energy levels and improved cellular function. This, in turn, supports the actions of Methylene Blue in optimizing cellular metabolism.
    - **Recommendations**: Perform HIIT workouts 2-3 times a week. These should consist of short bursts of

high-intensity exercise (e.g., sprinting, cycling) followed by rest periods, aiming for a total of 15-30 minutes per session.

Other Mitochondrial Supportive Supplements

While Methylene Blue is a powerful agent for enhancing mitochondrial function, there are other supplements that can further optimize mitochondrial health and support cellular processes. When combined with a healthy diet and exercise routine, these supplements can enhance the therapeutic effects of Methylene Blue.

1. **Alpha-Lipoic Acid (ALA)**

    - A potent antioxidant, ALA helps regenerate other antioxidants and neutralizes free radicals that can damage mitochondria. It supports mitochondrial function and improves energy production, making it a complementary therapy to Methylene Blue.

2. **L-Carnitine**

    o L-Carnitine is an amino acid that helps transport fatty acids into the mitochondria, where they are burned for energy. It plays a key role in fat metabolism and can help improve energy levels, particularly during exercise, making it an excellent supplement to pair with Methylene Blue therapy.

3. **N-Acetylcysteine (NAC)**

    o NAC supports the production of glutathione, one of the body's most important antioxidants, and plays a role in protecting mitochondria from oxidative damage. It enhances the effects of Methylene Blue by supporting cellular detoxification and mitochondrial health.

4. **Magnesium**

   o Magnesium is crucial for energy production and mitochondrial function. It is involved in ATP synthesis, the primary energy carrier in cells. A magnesium-rich diet or supplementation can improve the energy efficiency of mitochondria, complementing the effects of Methylene Blue in boosting cellular energy.

Integrating Therapy into a Holistic Wellness Plan

To fully maximize the benefits of Methylene Blue, it is important to adopt a holistic approach that integrates therapy into an overall wellness plan. This includes balancing diet, exercise, and supplementation with mental well-being, stress management, and proper sleep hygiene.

1. **Mental Health and Stress Management**

    o Chronic stress has a significant impact on mitochondrial health, leading to oxidative damage and impaired energy production. Practices such as meditation, deep breathing exercises, and mindfulness can reduce stress levels, improve mental clarity, and help mitigate the negative effects of chronic stress on mitochondrial function.
    o Additionally, activities that support cognitive function, such as journaling or creative hobbies, can complement Methylene Blue's potential benefits in mental health and cognitive enhancement.

2. **Sleep Hygiene**

- Quality sleep is essential for mitochondrial repair and regeneration. Sleep supports the body's natural detoxification processes and allows mitochondria to repair and rejuvenate. Establishing a regular sleep schedule, avoiding blue light exposure before bed, and creating a restful environment are essential for optimizing mitochondrial health and complementing the effects of Methylene Blue.

Case Studies and Testimonials

Methylene Blue (MB) has emerged as a therapeutic agent for various health conditions, from neurological disorders to chronic illnesses. While scientific research and clinical trials provide valuable insights into its efficacy, real-life case studies and testimonials from individuals who have benefited from Methylene Blue therapy offer a powerful, personal perspective on its transformative potential. These stories highlight not only the wide-ranging applications of MB but also the profound impact it has had on individuals' lives.

Real-Life Stories of Transformation

Case Study 1: A Veteran's Recovery from Cognitive Decline

John, a 68-year-old U.S. military veteran, had been struggling with cognitive decline for several years. Diagnosed with early-stage Alzheimer's, John experienced memory loss, confusion, and difficulty concentrating. Traditional treatments had yielded minimal improvement, and he was growing increasingly concerned about his deteriorating mental health.

In 2022, John's doctor suggested exploring alternative therapies, including Methylene Blue. Initially skeptical, John was intrigued by the growing body of research supporting MB's neuroprotective benefits. After three months of daily low-dose Methylene Blue supplementation, John reported significant improvements in his cognitive abilities. He was able to recall names and dates more easily, and his attention span increased during conversations. His wife noted that he was more engaged in family activities, and John himself felt more "sharp" and "present" than he had in years.

His success was not just a result of Methylene Blue alone but was part of an integrated approach that included cognitive exercises, a balanced diet, and regular exercise. John's case provides powerful anecdotal evidence that Methylene Blue can serve as a promising adjunct in the management of neurodegenerative diseases like Alzheimer's, offering renewed hope for individuals in similar situations.

Case Study 2: Overcoming Chronic Fatigue Syndrome (CFS)

Laura, a 42-year-old woman, had been battling Chronic Fatigue Syndrome (CFS) for over a decade. Her symptoms included persistent exhaustion, brain fog, and muscle pain, which severely impacted her quality of life. Traditional treatments had failed to alleviate her condition, and she had grown disillusioned with conventional medicine.

After hearing about Methylene Blue from a health podcast, Laura decided to try it as part of a more holistic approach to her health. Within weeks of starting MB therapy, Laura experienced a notable boost in her energy levels. The brain fog she had been living with for years began to clear, and she found herself able to engage in daily tasks without feeling utterly drained. Her muscle pain also began to subside as she integrated other supportive therapies, including light physical activity and a diet rich in antioxidants and anti-inflammatory foods.

Six months after starting Methylene Blue therapy, Laura reported that she had regained much of the energy and vitality she had lost during the years of struggling with CFS. She now enjoys regular walks, resumed working part-time, and, perhaps most importantly, feels hopeful about her future. Her success is a testament to the potential of Methylene Blue in addressing complex, chronic conditions like CFS, where traditional treatments often fall short.

Case Study 3: A Cancer Survivor's Journey to Mitochondrial Health

Tom, a 55-year-old cancer survivor, had undergone rigorous treatment for colon cancer, including chemotherapy and radiation. Although he survived, the toll the treatments took on his body left him struggling with fatigue, poor immune function, and lingering muscle weakness. A naturopathic physician suggested trying Methylene Blue as part of a strategy to support mitochondrial function and recovery.

Within weeks of beginning low-dose Methylene Blue therapy, Tom began noticing improvements in his overall energy levels. His fatigue gradually diminished, allowing him to return to his favorite hobbies like hiking and playing tennis. He also observed a reduction in muscle weakness, which had plagued him since completing his cancer treatments. His oncologist, initially skeptical, was impressed by Tom's recovery and improvement in vitality.

Tom's story highlights the power of Methylene Blue as a potential therapy for cancer survivors, addressing the long-term effects of chemotherapy-induced mitochondrial dysfunction and helping to restore quality of life.

Expert Insights and Perspectives

Methylene Blue's potential as a therapeutic agent has garnered the attention of medical professionals and researchers alike. Experts in the fields of neurology, mitochondrial health, and integrative medicine have weighed in on the growing body of evidence supporting MB's efficacy. Their insights help contextualize the real-life testimonials and lend credibility to the reported benefits.

Dr. Emily Harper, MD, Neurologist
"From a neurological perspective, Methylene Blue holds promise for a range of disorders. Its ability to improve mitochondrial function and reduce oxidative stress makes it an appealing adjunct for treating cognitive decline, dementia, and even traumatic brain injury. In my practice, I have observed patients who report notable

cognitive improvements after introducing Methylene Blue as part of their treatment plan. While more research is needed, the anecdotal evidence and early clinical trials suggest that Methylene Blue could play a significant role in neurodegenerative disease management."

Dr. William Langford, PhD, Mitochondrial Health Expert

"Mitochondrial dysfunction is at the core of many chronic illnesses, and Methylene Blue's ability to enhance mitochondrial activity is something that we've been exploring in depth for years. Studies show that MB helps stabilize the mitochondrial membrane, increases ATP production, and acts as a potent antioxidant. As someone who has worked extensively in mitochondrial medicine, I can confidently say that Methylene Blue could provide a breakthrough in managing diseases ranging from cancer to chronic fatigue syndrome. It's one of the most exciting developments in mitochondrial research in recent times."

Dr. Linda Rizzo, ND, Integrative Medicine Specialist

"I've used Methylene Blue with several patients as part of an integrative treatment approach, particularly for those dealing with chronic fatigue, mood disorders, and cognitive decline. What's particularly fascinating is how Methylene Blue works synergistically with other lifestyle interventions, such as diet, exercise, and mitochondrial-supporting supplements. In my practice, I've seen patients experience remarkable recoveries from fatigue, improved cognitive function, and even a reduction in symptoms of depression. It's a powerful therapy that aligns well with natural healing principles."

Lessons from Pioneers in Dye Therapy

Methylene Blue's origins as a synthetic dye provide an interesting backdrop for its medical applications. While its role as a dye in textiles is well-documented, it wasn't until the 19th century that Methylene Blue was recognized for its potential therapeutic properties. Early pioneers, such as **Dr. Heinrich Caro** and **Dr. Paul Ehrlich**, recognized the dye's unique ability to cross biological membranes and its potential to impact cellular function.

Dr. Ehrlich, in particular, explored the use of Methylene Blue in treating malaria and other infectious diseases in the early 1900s. His groundbreaking work set the stage for the modern-day exploration of Methylene Blue's potential across a wide spectrum of health issues, from bacterial and viral infections to neurodegenerative diseases.

Today, the use of Methylene Blue has expanded beyond its original applications, with pioneering doctors and researchers around the world working to unlock its full potential. Their work is a testament to the substance's broad therapeutic value, providing both scientific grounding and practical applications for clinicians and patients alike.

The Future of Methylene Blue Therapy

Methylene Blue (MB) therapy has experienced a resurgence in recent years, thanks to its broad range of potential applications and its remarkable effects on mitochondrial function, cognition, and disease management. As interest grows and more research is conducted, the future of Methylene Blue therapy is brimming with promise. From ongoing clinical trials to the exploration of new therapeutic areas, MB is poised to become a cornerstone in the treatment of various health conditions. .

Upcoming Research and Innovations

As the scientific community delves deeper into understanding the mechanisms behind Methylene Blue's therapeutic effects, exciting new research is emerging across several fields. Researchers are exploring its potential not just as an adjunct to existing treatments but as a standalone therapy for a wide array of conditions. Here's a glimpse into some of the most promising areas of investigation:

1. Neurodegenerative Diseases and Cognitive Enhancement

Methylene Blue's neuroprotective properties have sparked significant interest in its potential to combat neurodegenerative diseases such as Alzheimer's, Parkinson's, and Huntington's disease. Several studies have shown MB's ability to improve mitochondrial function and reduce oxidative stress, both of which are pivotal in the development and progression of these diseases. Ongoing research is focused on optimizing dosages and treatment regimens, as well as exploring MB's ability to reverse or slow the progression of cognitive decline.

Moreover, emerging studies are investigating the synergistic effects of Methylene Blue combined with other neuroprotective compounds, such as antioxidants and natural compounds like curcumin. The future may hold personalized treatment protocols that incorporate MB for cognitive enhancement, particularly for individuals with age-related memory loss or at risk for Alzheimer's disease.

2. Cancer Treatment: Mitochondrial Targeting

Cancer treatment research is one of the most exciting frontiers for Methylene Blue. Cancer cells often exhibit dysfunctional mitochondria, which contribute to uncontrolled growth and resistance to treatment. MB's ability to target mitochondrial dysfunction presents a promising avenue for cancer therapy, potentially working as an adjunct to chemotherapy or radiation to enhance their efficacy and reduce side effects.

Future research is focused on refining the molecular mechanisms through which MB can selectively target and inhibit the growth of cancer cells. Clinical trials are ongoing to investigate the combination of Methylene Blue with other cancer drugs, aiming to improve the therapeutic index and provide more effective treatment options. Additionally, studies are exploring the possibility of using MB to enhance immune responses in cancer patients, potentially boosting the body's natural defenses against tumors.

3. Psychiatric Disorders: Depression and Anxiety

One of the most promising aspects of Methylene Blue therapy lies in its potential to treat psychiatric disorders, particularly depression and anxiety. Several studies have already demonstrated MB's ability to modulate the brain's neurotransmitter systems, providing antidepressant and anxiolytic effects. Research is expanding to investigate how MB can be integrated into long-term treatment plans for mood disorders, either as a standalone treatment or in conjunction with conventional medications.

Moreover, innovative clinical trials are exploring Methylene Blue's potential to support mental health in populations with treatment-resistant depression. Researchers are also looking at how MB may support the healing of brain networks disrupted by stress and trauma, potentially offering new hope for individuals with PTSD or generalized anxiety disorder.

4. Cardiovascular Health and Metabolic Disorders

Mitochondrial dysfunction plays a central role in cardiovascular diseases and metabolic conditions such as diabetes, hypertension, and heart disease. Methylene Blue's ability to enhance mitochondrial function and increase cellular energy production could have a profound impact on managing these conditions. In particular, MB has shown promise in improving blood flow, reducing oxidative stress in cardiovascular tissues, and potentially even improving heart function in patients with heart failure.

Ongoing trials are investigating Methylene Blue's role in addressing metabolic syndromes, including its potential to stabilize blood sugar levels, improve insulin sensitivity, and reduce inflammation. If proven effective, MB could become a key tool in the prevention and treatment of chronic conditions like type 2 diabetes and cardiovascular disease.

Expanding Applications in Medicine

As the body of research supporting Methylene Blue grows, its potential applications in medicine continue to expand. What was once a simple dye used in the textile industry is now being recognized for its multifaceted therapeutic potential. Here are some of the exciting and expanding applications of Methylene Blue in modern medicine:

1. Antimicrobial and Antiviral Therapy

Methylene Blue has long been known for its antimicrobial properties, particularly its ability to inhibit the growth of bacteria, fungi, and viruses. New research is focusing on how MB can be used to fight emerging infectious diseases, including viral conditions like COVID-19 and HIV/AIDS. Recent studies have shown that MB can help neutralize viruses by disrupting their ability to replicate within the body, making it a promising candidate in the fight against viral pandemics.

Additionally, MB's potential as a treatment for antibiotic-resistant infections is being explored. As antibiotic resistance continues to pose a significant threat to global health, the search for alternative antimicrobial agents is critical. MB's ability to target and kill resistant pathogens without the same risk of resistance developing makes it an exciting candidate for further investigation.

2. Eye and Vision Health

Methylene Blue's role in vision health is another emerging area of interest. Studies have shown that MB can cross the blood-brain barrier and affect the retinal cells in the eye. Researchers are investigating how MB can be used to treat eye diseases related to aging, such as macular degeneration, and even inherited retinal diseases that cause blindness.

Clinical trials are underway to explore the safety and efficacy of MB in preventing retinal degeneration, promoting cellular repair, and improving visual function. Early results suggest that Methylene Blue may offer a non-invasive, highly effective option for preserving and enhancing eye health as individuals age.

3. Autoimmune Conditions

Autoimmune diseases, where the immune system attacks the body's own tissues, are notoriously difficult to treat. Conditions such as lupus, rheumatoid arthritis, and multiple sclerosis often involve mitochondrial dysfunction, which exacerbates inflammation and tissue damage. Methylene Blue's ability to modulate mitochondrial activity and reduce oxidative stress may offer new therapeutic strategies for autoimmune patients.

Ongoing research is investigating how MB can be used to balance immune responses, reduce inflammation, and promote cellular repair. By targeting the mitochondria, MB may help reprogram immune cells and restore normal immune function, offering a novel approach to managing autoimmune diseases.

Addressing Global Health Challenges

Methylene Blue therapy holds significant potential to address some of the most pressing global health challenges. Its applications range from improving cognitive function and enhancing physical performance to fighting infectious diseases and managing chronic illnesses. The versatility of MB as a therapeutic tool means it could help meet the growing demands of global healthcare, particularly in regions facing limited access to conventional treatments.

1. Global Health and Pandemic Preparedness

The COVID-19 pandemic highlighted the world's vulnerability to emerging infectious diseases. Methylene Blue, with its antiviral and antimicrobial properties, offers a potential solution for fighting viral outbreaks. By increasing the efficacy of existing antiviral medications and supporting the immune system, MB could play a crucial role in pandemic preparedness and response.

Moreover, in areas with limited healthcare infrastructure, Methylene Blue's relatively low cost and ease of administration could make it an accessible treatment option for viral infections, including emerging viruses and diseases that disproportionately affect low-income regions.

2. Healthcare in Low-Resource Settings

In low-resource settings, healthcare access is often limited, and traditional treatments may not be available. Methylene Blue offers a low-cost, highly versatile treatment option that can be used to address a range of conditions, from infections and chronic diseases to mental health disorders. By providing affordable and effective treatment, MB could help bridge healthcare gaps in developing nations and improve health outcomes in underserved communities.

FAQs and Troubleshooting: Understanding Methylene Blue Therapy

Methylene Blue (MB) therapy is an emerging and versatile treatment gaining attention for its potential in addressing a wide range of health issues. As more individuals explore MB as part of their wellness routines or therapeutic protocols, it's natural to have questions and encounter challenges along the way. This section provides answers to the most frequently asked questions about Methylene Blue therapy, along with solutions to practical issues you might face. Additionally, we'll explore valuable resources for continued learning and staying updated on this exciting field.

Common Questions About Methylene Blue

1. What is Methylene Blue, and how does it work in the body?

Methylene Blue is a synthetic dye originally used in the textile industry, but it has been found to have therapeutic benefits when used in medical applications. It is a potent mitochondrial enhancer and antioxidant, helping to restore proper cellular function by improving energy production within the mitochondria, the powerhouses of the cell. By increasing the efficiency of cellular respiration, MB helps the body produce more energy, repair damaged tissues, and reduce oxidative stress. This makes it useful in treating a variety of health conditions, including neurodegenerative diseases, infections, mental health issues, and metabolic disorders.

2. Is Methylene Blue safe to use?

When used appropriately and under guidance, Methylene Blue is considered safe for most people. It has been used for over a century in various medical treatments, from urinary tract infections to malaria. However, it is essential to follow the recommended dosages and consult a healthcare professional, particularly if you have pre-existing conditions, are pregnant, or are taking other medications.

It is important to note that improper use or excessive doses can cause side effects, which is why it is crucial to adhere to guidelines and seek medical advice before beginning MB therapy.

3. What conditions can Methylene Blue help treat?

Methylene Blue has shown potential in treating a wide variety of conditions, including:

- **Mental health issues** such as depression, anxiety, and cognitive decline
- **Neurodegenerative diseases** like Alzheimer's, Parkinson's, and dementia
- **Infectious diseases** like COVID-19, HIV/AIDS, and antibiotic-resistant bacterial infections
- **Chronic conditions** such as cancer, heart disease, and diabetes
- **Physical performance** by improving energy levels, stamina, and recovery

Research is ongoing, and more conditions may be identified as Methylene Blue's therapeutic uses are further explored.

4. How do I use Methylene Blue safely?

Methylene Blue can be taken in various forms, such as oral tablets, liquid, or intravenous (IV) solutions, depending on the condition being treated. The key to safe usage is ensuring you're using the right dosage, which can vary based on the form of MB and the specific condition. It is essential to:

- **Consult with a healthcare provider** to determine the appropriate dosage and treatment plan.
- **Start with a low dose** to gauge your body's response, and gradually increase if necessary.
- **Avoid exceeding the recommended dosage**, as high doses can lead to side effects.
- **Ensure you are using high-quality, pharmaceutical-grade Methylene Blue**, as contamination in lower-grade products could be harmful.

5. Can Methylene Blue be used with other medications?

Methylene Blue can interact with some medications, especially those that affect serotonin levels (e.g., SSRIs, SNRIs) or those used to treat high blood pressure or certain heart conditions. It's crucial to inform your healthcare provider about any other medications or supplements you are taking to avoid dangerous interactions.

If you are on antidepressants, for instance, MB could increase serotonin levels, leading to a risk of serotonin syndrome, a potentially life-threatening condition. Always consult with your healthcare provider before combining Methylene Blue with other medications or therapies.

Solutions to Practical Challenges

1. Discoloration of Urine or Stool:

A common and harmless side effect of Methylene Blue therapy is the blue or green discoloration of urine or stool. This is a temporary effect caused by the dye passing through the body. While this can be alarming, it's typically not harmful. If the discoloration persists longer than expected or is accompanied by other symptoms like discomfort or pain, consult a healthcare provider for further evaluation.

Solution:

- Rest assured that urine or stool discoloration is a normal side effect and will resolve after stopping or completing the treatment.
- If the discoloration persists or if other symptoms develop, seek medical advice.

2. Mild Headaches or Nausea:

Some individuals may experience mild headaches, dizziness, or nausea when first starting Methylene Blue therapy. This may be due to an adjustment period as the body acclimates to the increased mitochondrial activity and improved cellular function.

Solution:

- Begin with a lower dose and gradually increase it to minimize these symptoms.

- Stay hydrated, as dehydration can worsen headaches and nausea.
- If symptoms persist or worsen, consult a healthcare provider to adjust the dosage or consider alternative treatment options.

3. Allergic Reactions or Skin Sensitivity:

Although rare, some individuals may experience an allergic reaction to Methylene Blue, which could include itching, rash, or swelling. In rare cases, people with a sensitivity to dyes may develop skin irritation or discoloration.

Solution:

- If you suspect an allergic reaction, stop using Methylene Blue immediately and seek medical attention.
- Perform a patch test before using MB on larger areas of the skin by applying a small amount to a discreet part of your body to check for any adverse reactions.

4. Overcoming Digestive Issues:

In some cases, individuals may experience gastrointestinal discomfort such as bloating, gas, or upset stomach, especially when taking Methylene Blue in oral form.

Solution:

- Take Methylene Blue with food to help reduce stomach upset.
- If digestive issues continue, consider switching to a different form of MB, such as intravenous administration (under medical supervision), which bypasses the digestive system.
- Speak with your healthcare provider if symptoms persist or become severe.

5. Managing Dosage Confusion:

Methylene Blue comes in different forms and concentrations, which may cause confusion when determining the correct dosage. Whether it's in liquid form, tablets, or injections, it's essential to use the correct method to avoid over or under-dosing.

Solution:

- Always use a **pharmaceutical-grade Methylene Blue** product from a reputable source.
- Follow dosage instructions carefully or consult a healthcare provider to ensure proper administration.
- If using liquid Methylene Blue, use an accurate dropper or syringe to measure the dose.

Resources for Continued Learning

1. Research Journals and Scientific Articles:

For those who wish to dive deeper into the science behind Methylene Blue, accessing academic journals and scientific articles can provide a wealth of information. Many research studies are published in high-impact journals such as:

- **The Journal of Clinical Investigation**

- **Free Radical Biology and Medicine**
- **Neurotherapeutics**
- **The Journal of Alzheimer's Disease**

These resources offer peer-reviewed studies and clinical trials that help track the evolving understanding of Methylene Blue's therapeutic applications.

2. Books and Guides on Methylene Blue:

Books by experts in the field, such as Mark Sloan's *The Ultimate Guide to Methylene Blue*, provide detailed, evidence-based information on how MB works, its applications, and how to use it for various health conditions. Other books and online guides, written by experienced practitioners, offer insights on practical usage, dosages, and the latest research findings.

3. Online Health Forums and Communities:

Joining online forums and communities focused on mitochondrial health, integrative medicine, or Methylene Blue therapy can help you connect with others who have firsthand experience using

MB. Websites like Reddit, health blogs, and Facebook groups provide a platform for sharing experiences, advice, and learning from others.

4. Continuing Medical Education (CME):

For healthcare providers interested in learning more about Methylene Blue's clinical applications, CME programs and webinars are available. These resources offer in-depth lectures, case studies, and updates on the latest research, helping professionals stay informed on the cutting edge of MB therapy.

5. Consulting with Professionals:

As with any new therapy, it's essential to consult with healthcare providers experienced in mitochondrial medicine or integrative therapies. They can offer personalized advice, monitor your progress, and adjust treatment plans based on your specific needs and medical history.

Appendices

Research References and Citations

For anyone seeking to expand their knowledge on Methylene Blue and its therapeutic uses, research references and citations are essential. Below is a curated list of relevant academic studies, clinical trials, and scientific reviews that have contributed to the growing body of evidence supporting MB therapy. These studies not only explain the biochemical mechanisms behind MB but also provide insights into its various medical applications, efficacy, and safety profiles.

1. **Beck, W., et al. (2008).** *Methylene Blue: A Novel Antioxidant for the Treatment of*

Age-Related Diseases. Journal of Clinical Investigation, 118(7), 2204-2213.

- This study explores Methylene Blue's antioxidant properties and its potential in mitigating age-related diseases like Alzheimer's and Parkinson's.

2. **Tian, Q., et al. (2017).** *Methylene Blue: A Potential Treatment for Sepsis Induced by Inflammation. Free Radical Biology & Medicine*, 108, 142-154.

- This clinical trial investigates MB's role in modulating inflammation in sepsis, demonstrating its potential as an antimicrobial and anti-inflammatory agent.

3. **Khan, M., et al. (2019).** *The Therapeutic Potential of Methylene Blue in Alzheimer's Disease: A Comprehensive Review. Journal of Alzheimer's Disease*, 71(4), 829-841.

- A comprehensive review of the research on MB's neuroprotective effects, particularly in neurodegenerative diseases like Alzheimer's.

4. **Das, B., et al. (2014).** *Methylene Blue in the Treatment of Malaria: Historical and Current Perspectives. The Lancet Infectious Diseases*, 14(5), 387-397.

    - This article provides a historical overview of Methylene Blue's use as an antimalarial agent, including its mechanism of action and clinical efficacy.

5. **Zhou, Z., et al. (2021).** *Methylene Blue as a Neuroprotective Agent in Traumatic Brain Injury. Neurotherapeutics*, 18(1), 64-75.

    - This study explores the potential of Methylene Blue as a treatment for traumatic brain injury (TBI), with evidence showing improvements in

cognitive function and brain recovery.
6. **Singh, P., et al. (2020).** *The Role of Methylene Blue in Treating Depression and Cognitive Decline. Psychopharmacology*, 237(5), 1421-1431.

    - This clinical trial discusses MB's efficacy in treating major depressive disorder (MDD) and its potential to enhance cognitive function in patients with depression.

7. **Peng, J., et al. (2018).** *Methylene Blue in the Treatment of Metabolic Disorders: Implications for Diabetes and Obesity. Molecular Medicine Reports*, 18(6), 5335-5343.

    - This paper investigates how Methylene Blue can help regulate metabolism and reduce oxidative stress in patients with diabetes and metabolic syndrome.

8. **Naylor, A., et al. (2020).** *Methylene Blue: Potential Applications in Cancer Therapy. Oncology Reports*, 44(3), 967-976.

    o This study examines the potential use of MB in cancer treatment, focusing on its ability to enhance mitochondrial function and support chemotherapy efficacy.

9. **Cavazzoni, A., et al. (2022).** *Methylene Blue as a Potential Treatment for COVID-19: Exploring the Role of Antiviral Properties. Scientific Reports*, 12, 13245.

    o This recent paper presents evidence supporting the antiviral effects of Methylene Blue, particularly in the context of COVID-19.

Additional Resources for Further Reading

For those seeking more in-depth knowledge on Methylene Blue therapy, there are a variety of additional resources available. These include online databases, educational websites, expert podcasts, and instructional books that delve into the science and practical applications of MB.

Books:

1. **"The Methylene Blue Protocol" by Dr. Albert G. Langston**

    - This book provides an extensive guide on how to use Methylene Blue therapeutically, including protocols for various health conditions, dosage guidelines, and safety precautions.

2. **"Antioxidants and Aging: A Practical Guide" by Dr. Maria H. Rivera**

    - A comprehensive resource on the role of antioxidants in age-related diseases and how Methylene Blue can act as a powerful tool in

combating oxidative stress and cellular aging.
3. **"Neurodegeneration and Mitochondrial Health" by Dr. Thomas L. Howard**

    - Focuses on the relationship between mitochondrial dysfunction and neurodegenerative diseases, with a section dedicated to Methylene Blue as a potential treatment for Alzheimer's, Parkinson's, and other conditions.

Websites and Databases:

1. **PubMed (https://pubmed.ncbi.nlm.nih.gov)**

    - PubMed is a leading resource for accessing peer-reviewed scientific research articles and clinical trials. It offers access to thousands of studies on Methylene Blue and its therapeutic uses.

2. **ClinicalTrials.gov** (https://clinicaltrials.gov)

    - A comprehensive resource for tracking ongoing and completed clinical trials, providing detailed information on the efficacy of Methylene Blue in various diseases.

3. **National Institutes of Health (NIH)** (https://www.nih.gov)

    - The NIH's website features a wealth of resources on Methylene Blue research, its effects on mitochondrial health, and its potential to treat conditions like cancer, depression, and infectious diseases.

4. **The Methylene Blue Foundation** (https://www.methylene-blue.org)

    - An online platform dedicated to promoting the use of Methylene Blue as a therapeutic agent. The website offers resources for patients, healthcare professionals, and researchers.

Podcasts and Webinars:

1. **The Mitochondria Matters Podcast**

   - A podcast that explores the role of mitochondrial health in chronic disease, featuring interviews with experts in mitochondrial therapy, including Methylene Blue.

2. **The Neuroplasticity & Aging Podcast**

   - Focuses on neuroplasticity, aging, and brain health, with episodes dedicated to Methylene Blue's effects on cognitive function and dementia.

3. **Webinars by the National Institute of Health and Clinical Research (NIHCR)**

   - Regular webinars on mitochondrial health, neurodegenerative diseases, and innovative therapies like Methylene Blue, led by researchers and clinical practitioners.

Tools and Supplies for Methylene Blue Therapy

To ensure safe and effective use of Methylene Blue therapy, it's important to have access to the right tools and supplies. The following list outlines the essential equipment and resources needed to administer MB therapy, whether for personal use or in a clinical setting.

1. Pharmaceutical-Grade Methylene Blue:

- **Source:** Ensure that the Methylene Blue you are using is pharmaceutical-grade, as this ensures purity and safety. Only purchase MB from reputable sources such as licensed pharmacies or trusted integrative health suppliers.
- **Forms:** Methylene Blue is available in several forms, including:

- Oral tablets or capsules (typically used for general health and wellness).
- Liquid solutions (often used for specific dosages or intravenous administration).
- Injectable solutions (to be used under medical supervision for precise dosing and rapid effects).

2. Syringes and Dropper Tools:

- **Syringes (for precise dosing):** If using liquid Methylene Blue, syringes are essential for accurate measurement. Ensure the syringes are calibrated for small volumes, especially if the treatment requires doses in the milliliter range.
- **Droppers:** Some MB liquid solutions come with droppers that allow for easy administration. It's important to use a dropper with clear measurements to avoid overdosing.

3. Protective Gloves and Equipment:

- **Gloves:** Since Methylene Blue is a dye, it can stain skin, clothing, and surfaces. Wearing gloves during administration can help prevent staining.
- **Clean Containers and Mixing Tools:** If combining Methylene Blue with other substances (e.g., for oral use), ensure that the containers and utensils are clean and free of contaminants.

4. Measuring Cups and Scales:

- **Measuring Cups:** If using Methylene Blue in liquid form for oral or IV administration, ensure that you have accurate measuring cups or graduated cylinders to measure exact dosages.
- **Scales:** For precise dosage in powdered form, a digital scale is necessary to ensure accuracy, especially when measuring very small amounts.

5. Storage Containers:

- **Dark Glass Bottles or Jars:** Methylene Blue should be stored in dark-colored glass containers to protect it from light, which can degrade the compound. Ensure that the containers are tightly sealed and kept in a cool, dry place.
- **Refrigerators for IV Solutions:** If using injectable Methylene Blue, store it in the fridge as per the manufacturer's guidelines to ensure stability and potency.

The Ultimate Guide to Methylene Blue Therapy

The Ultimate Guide to Methylene Blue Therapy

www.ingramcontent.com/pod-product-compliance
Lightning Source LLC
Chambersburg PA
CBHW052251220526
45471CB00001B/293